Rudolf Steiner and Holistic Medicine

Rudolf Steiner and Holistic Medicine

Francis X. King

NICOLAS-HAYS, INC.
York Beach, Maine

First published in the United States of America in 1987 by
Nicolas-Hays, Inc.
Box 612
York Beach, Maine 03910

Reprinted, 1991

Distributed to the trade by
Samuel Weiser, Inc.
Box 612
York Beach, Maine 03910

Library of Congress Cataloging in Publication Data:
    King, Francis X.
        Rudolf Steiner and holistic medicine.

        Originally published: London : Rider, 1986.
        Bibliography: p.
            1. Anthroposophical therapy.   2. Holistic medicine.
    I. Steiner, Rudolf, 1861–1925.   II. Title. [DNLM:
    1. Holistic Health. W 61 K52r]
    RZ409.7.K56   1987   610   87-12290

ISBN 0-89254-015-X
BJ

Cover photograph © Phillip Augusta. Used by kind permission.

Printed in the United States of America

CONTENTS

6 *Contents*

PART ONE

Rudolf Steiner and Anthroposophical Medicine

1

Holistic Medicine and Rudolf Steiner

'Be no longer a drinker of water, but use a little wine for thy stomach's sake and thine often infirmities.' Such, almost two thousand years ago, was the advice given by St Paul, tentmaker turned evangelist, to Timothy. Ever since then the medically unqualified have been unsparing in the advice they have given one another on the subjects of health and sickness.

In the last ten years or so such advice has tended to be concerned with what is usually designated as either 'alternative' or 'complementary' medicine. At social gatherings friends and acquaintances urge one another to have backache treated by chiropractors or osteopaths, to give up smoking with the aid of traditional Chinese acupuncture, to take homoeopathic prophylactics for hayfever and other allergies, and even to induce mood changes by the use of aromatherapy. All those who practise these and other unorthodox therapies, such as nature cure and traditional herbalism, consider themselves to be involved in 'holistic medicine'; that is, they aver that they are treating the whole human being, not some particular part of him or her.

'Holistic' is a comparatively new adjective, derived from the word 'holism', which General Smuts coined sixty years ago as a description of his philosophical belief that the fundamental principle of the cosmos is the creation of 'wholes', i.e. self-contained systems of lesser or greater complexity. While the phrase 'holistic medicine' is thus a very new one, the idea that is intended to be conveyed by it, that a therapist should endeavour to treat the whole human being, is far from new. It underlies the Ayurvedic medicine which has been derived from ancient India, the traditional herbalism, acupuncture and moxibustion of China, and such Western medical unorthodoxies as naturopathy and homoeopathy.

At the root of all these therapeutic systems can be discerned the same basic premises: that the totally healthy human organism which is functioning as it should be either does not become ill or, if it does suffer sickness, makes a rapid spontaneous recovery, and that the occurrence of any illness, even one which seems confined to a particular organ, indicates that there is something wrong with the functioning of the patient's mind and body *as a whole*.

The treatment administered by Chinese acupuncturists illustrates this approach, with needles sometimes being inserted into the body at positions so far removed from the site at which a disease is manifesting itself that in the past some European travellers came to the mistaken conclusion that they were inserted at random. In reality, of course, the acupuncturist uses a highly schematized theoretical framework in order to select particular points to stimulate, either by the insertion of needles or the application of smouldering cones of dried mugwort leaves, with the object of restoring to normal the subtle energy flows which are believed to control the functioning of mind and body. Whether or not such energy flows actually exist is a matter for debate; the essential point is that the practitioner of acupuncture who is the master of his art is not following some empirical set of rules, such as 'if the patient has a headache insert needles at points A, B and C', but is making a separate clinical judgement at each individual consultation, deciding what measures may be applicable to a particular patient for the purpose of restoring his or her total functioning to normality. Thus two patients who come to an acupuncturist with the same complaint – hayfever, for example – would be treated by quite different patterns of point stimulation if the practitioner decided, on the basis of traditional diagnostic techniques and clinical judgement, that different sorts of interruption of energy flows had resulted in very similar physical symptoms. In the words of a phrase which is commonly used by many practitioners of alternative and complementary medicine, the acupuncturist is 'treating the patient, not the disease'.

An even more patient-orientated system of diagnosis and remedy selection characterizes homoeopathy, which, with the exception of traditional herbalism, is the oldest Western system of holistic therapy, its origins probably going back as far as the sixteenth century. For although it was not until around the beginning of the last century that Samuel Hahnemann (1755–1843) gave the first full exposition of homoeopathic theory and practice, its fundamental principles – that 'like cures like', that a patient should be treated by very small doses of substances which in large doses produce effects similar to the symptoms of that patient's disease – can be found expressed in much older texts. Thus, for example, precisely the same Latin phrase which Hahnemann used to express the core of his teachings, *similia similibus curantur* ('like cures like'), can be found as the heading of a paragraph in the 1658 edition of the *Works* of Paracelsus, the sixteenth-century alchemist, mystic and healer.

In some ways Hahnemann's greatest achievement was not his theory, but the way in which he worked, the example he gave of how the search for a remedy should be undertaken. Like Goethe, he believed that 'the phenomena should be the doctrine'. In other words, he believed that the healer must act in accordance with what is actually perceived in both nature and the individual patient, not on the basis of preconceived empirical notions. 'Empirical' is here used not in its philosophical but in its medical sense as a description of the anti-Hippocratic school of therapy which originated in Greece and the influence of which has survived until the present day.

In accordance with his Goethe-like approach, Hahnemann sought his remedies by 'proving' plant, animal and mineral substances on healthy volunteers, administering steadily increasing doses until symptoms similar to those of disease were produced in his subjects. The substances in question were then subjected to extreme dilution and administered to patients whose symptoms were similar to those produced by large doses of the undiluted remedy.

The results reported were often very remarkable indeed. Patients with chronic complaints, against which the orthodox remedies of the time had proved powerless, were cured or their condition was greatly improved, while in cases of severe infection the recovery rate of those treated with Hahnemann's medicines was far better than that of those prescribed orthodox remedies.

Homoeopathy has not stood still in the 125 years or so since Samuel Hahnemann's death, and a large number of remedies have since then been added to the homoeopathic therapeutic armoury; it seems probable that a substantial, though unquantifiable, proportion of these has come into use as a result of accumulated clinical experience rather than individual 'provings'.

That this is indeed the case would seem to be confirmed by a research report recently published in the *British Homoeopathic Journal*. Three widely used homoeopathic remedies – arnica, bryonia and pulsatilla – were administered in steadily increasing dose to seven volunteers, four men and three women, all of them qualified physicians. The trial was a 'double blind': neither the volunteers who took the remedies nor the physician administering them were aware of their nature. In fairly substantial doses two of the remedies, arnica and bryonia, did not produce in any of the volunteers symptoms similar to those of the diseases for which, in dilute form, they are prescribed. The third remedy, pulsatilla, widely prescribed as a homoeopathic remedy for premenstrual abdominal pains, produced similar symptoms in only one of the women volunteers; in view of the smallness of the sample no statistical significance could be attached to this. In spite of this negative result, however, the fact remains that literally millions of patients have found that on a purely pragmatic basis, quite regardless of theories concerning 'like cures like', homoeopathy has worked *for them*.

Over the decades the popularity of homoeopathy has waxed, waned and waxed again. It has always, however, retained a certain following and in Britain has sometimes been regarded as the Establishment's alternative medicine – for over a century the royal family have had a homoeopathic physician amongst their medical attendants and, perhaps as a result of this, homoeopathy has always been incorporated into the National Health Service. In recent years there has been something of a European revival of interest in homoeopathic medicine and this has led to suggestions by orthodox practitioners that a series of comparative trials of conventional and homoeopathic remedies should be carried out under the usual 'double blind' test conditions. Such suggestions may indicate an increasing disquiet amongst medical practitioners about both the increasing popularity of alternative medicine and the alarming incidence of iatrogenic disorders, that is, illness actually caused by the drugs administered to patients. They also indicate, however, a lack of awareness of how holistic practitioners in general and homoeopathic physicians in particular prescribe for their patients.

There is no one drug, or even one of a baker's dozen or so of drugs, which a homoeopathic physician will invariably prescribe as, say, a sedative or a prophylactic against hayfever. The prescription will be tailored to fit the particular patient, not his or her complaint, and the homoeopathic practitioner may refer to an individual as 'the such-and-such a remedy type', meaning that the psychophysical make-up of that patient has been diagnosed as being of such a nature that it will respond particularly well to a particular drug *which may be considered as being totally unsuitable for another patient suffering from the same complaint.*

A variant of this, the same remedy being prescribed to two different patients for seemingly unrelated complaints – for example, heart disease and manic outbursts of fury – is sometimes a feature of a system of holistic therapy which has undoubtedly been much influenced by certain aspects of homoeopathy. This is anthroposophical medicine, which, unlike acupuncture or homoeopathy, is only rarely the subject of conversational chitchat in the English-speaking world. The adjectives 'anthroposophical' and 'anthroposophic' are , of course, derived from the noun 'anthroposophy'.[1] In the past this noun and words derived from it were sometimes used in a pejorative sense – thus in Charles Kingsley's novel *Yeast* the word 'anthroposophist' implies someone who followed human rather than divine wisdom –

but in current usage it means 'the understanding of the inmost, spiritual nature of man'.

The main reason why anthroposophical therapies are rarely discussed (apart from the difficulty some of us experience in pronouncing the word 'anthroposophical') is that only a small minority of Americans and Britons are even vaguely aware of the existence of anthroposophical medicine and its practitioners. In continental Europe, particularly in Germany, Holland and Switzerland, the number of anthroposophical physicians and surgeons is much greater. Thus in Germany, for example, there are eleven hospitals, one of them specializing in psychiatry, in which anthroposophical medicine is practised.

In such hospitals the approach is, of course, holistic, its aim being to treat the patient not the disease. Not only are conventional medicaments prescribed – although much less frequently in the case of antibiotics – but also homoeopathic and specifically anthroposophic remedies. In addition, many patients receive various types of massage, medicinal baths, and even instruction in painting and a therapeutic variety of the art of movement known as eurhythmy. These and other therapeutic techniques make up that extension of the art of healing which those who practise anthroposophical medicine believe it to be.

Anthroposophical medicine had its origins in the teachings of Rudolf Steiner (1861–1925), the Austrian scholar, philosopher and mystic, and is usually considered to have only really begun to be formulated in 1920, when Steiner delivered his first course of lectures specifically aimed at a medical audience. As is explained in Appendix I, there are reasons to believe that some form of complementary medicine based on indications given by Steiner was, in fact, being practised by medically qualified students of his teachings well before the outbreak of the 1914–18 war. Nevertheless, it is undoubted that there was no real awareness of the existence of anthroposophical medicine, even amongst that minority inclined to the use of alternative and complementary therapies, until the very last years of Steiner's life. This does not mean that the earlier years of Rudolf Steiner's life, the years in which he developed both his philosophy and, according to his pupils, certain higher faculties of perception, are devoid of significance for the student of holistic medicine – quite the contrary. Anthroposophical medicine is perhaps the most holistic of all philosophies of healing, for it is not just concerned with the whole body as a unity, or even with body and mind as a unified and self-contained biosystem, but with body, mind and spirit, the *soma, psyche* and *pneuma* of the New Testament's Greek original. This approach is not confined to the anthroposophical extension of healing; it characterizes the similar extensions of, for example, education, agriculture, art and architecture, and is almost entirely derived from the intellectual and spiritual concepts which Rudolf Steiner developed in comparatively early life. This development cannot be wholly understood without some knowledge of the most important events of Steiner's life.

Rudolf Steiner was born in 1861 at Kraljevic, a small town then on the eastern borders of the Austro-Hungarian Empire and now part of Yugoslavia. His father was a minor employee of the South Austrian region of the Royal and Imperial Railways and hoped that one day his son would also become a railwayman – perhaps, hoped Herr Steiner, an engineer. To this end it was decided that the young Rudolf should not attend a *Gymnasium*, a school in which much emphasis was placed on the importance of classical learning, but a *Realschule*, roughly the equivalent of an English technical school.

The *Realschule* was succeeded by the Viennese *Technische Hochschule*, literally a 'technical high school', but in status more nearly resembling a university which specialized in engineering and allied subjects but also insisted upon its students acquiring some knowledge of their native literature. Steiner flourished in this intellectual environment; even as a child he had found poetry as absorbing as mathematics. Indeed, for the young Steiner mathematics was, in a sense, poetry – he had found the demonstrations of Euclidean geometry to be *beautiful* as well as intellectually satisfying.

The Professor of German Literary History at the *Hochschule* was Karl Julius Schroer, a man who profoundly influenced the course of Steiner's life by, first, firing him with enthusiasm for the holistic philosophy of science which had been developed by Goethe; secondly, by obtaining jobs for him; and, lastly, by introducing him to some of the artists, writers, musicians and dilettante intellectuals who frequented the Griensteidl Kaffee. This latter establishment was sarcastically nicknamed 'the Megalomania Café', but was nevertheless the centre of avant-garde intellectualism in the Vienna of the 1880s. Schroer seems to have been both intrigued and impressed by Steiner's admiration for Goethe's scientific writings – at the time, as now, they were generally regarded as, at best, the eccentric by-products of poetic genius – and induced the publishers of a vast compendium of over 200 volumes entitled *German National Literature* to allow the young man to edit those works of Goethe concerned with biology and physics.

The work was satisfying but ill-paid, and Steiner supplemented his income by tutorial work, cramming slow-witted or lazy children for the various public examinations which were such an important feature of the Austrian educational system. One such tutorial experience was to prove of considerable importance in the development of Steiner's theories concerning 'curative education', an integral part of what is now known as anthroposophical medicine.

A certain Herr Specht, an acquaintance of Karl Schroer, had a ten-year-old son, Otto, who was supposedly mentally retarded, his backwardness attributed to hydrocephaly, water on the brain. Steiner came to the conclusion that there was nothing fundamentally wrong with the boy's mind; the real cause of the seeming mental retardation was that the undeveloped body was not working in harmony with the mind – to use an analogy from mechanical engineering, it was as though the fault was in the transmission, not the engine. What was needed, decided Steiner, was to give the boy what old-fashioned teachers termed 'mental confidence'. This, so he believed, would result in Otto's mind and body working together in harmony, as nature, in the full Goethean sense of the word, intended.

Steiner's confidence-inducing teaching was spectacularly successful. Within two years or so the 'mentally retarded' Otto had caught up with his contemporaries and passed the entrance examination which admitted him to the

Gymnasium. The mental changes were accompanied by physical changes, the hydrocephaly steadily diminishing. This surprised Steiner, and led him to the conclusion (now generally accepted but then highly unorthodox) that the state of the mind can be productive of physical changes in the human organism. Subsequently Otto Specht qualified as a medical practitioner and served in the Austrian army during the First World War.

At this period of his life Rudolf Steiner was not a student of occultism in the full sense of those words. Nevertheless, he was not unacquainted with occult theories, for amongst those he knew as frequenters of the Megalomania Café were a number of students of esotericism, oriental religion and mystical philosophy. The most notable of these was Friedrich Eckstein, a wealthy paper manufacturer who had become captivated by the Theosophy of Madame Blavatsky and her closest associates – Colonel Olcott, A. P. Sinnett and the dubious occultist Dr Franz Hartmann. Just how great was Eckstein's devotion to Theosophy is shown by the fact that for a full year he endured having the unpleasant Hartmann, 'dirty Franz', so-called because of his personal habits, as his non-paying guest.

Eckstein had a wide circle of acquaintances[2] and introduced Steiner to most of the leading figures in the Vienna Lodge of the Theosophical Society. On the whole, however, Steiner was not impressed by Theosophy and the occult theories associated with it, finding the latter alien and even repellent. He seems to have particularly disliked A. P. Sinnett's book *Esoteric Buddhism*, a copy of which had been lent him by Eckstein. In spite of its title, *Esoteric Buddhism*, an occult best seller of the 1880s, was in no way concerned with Buddhism, either esoteric or otherwise. It was a first formulation, based on letters which Sinnett had allegedly received from the Mahatmas, supposed superhuman beings who were believed to live in Tibet, of the remarkable system of occult cosmology and history which found full expression in Madame Blavatsky's *Secret Doctrine*.

What repelled Rudolf Steiner about Theosophical literature in general and *Esoteric Buddhism* in particular was what he considered to be its underlying hostility – usually implicit but sometimes explicit – to the traditions of mystical Christianity. In a lecture given almost thirty years after he had first read Sinnett's book he affirmed that:

The greatest mistake of the Theosophical Society was first made by Madame H. P. Blavatsky. For . . . in the contents of her upper consciousness, in her wishes and desires, there was a continuing antipathy, even a passion, against all things Jewish or Christian, and a preference for every other spiritual culture . . . she conceived of Christ in a totally false manner. . . . Her attitude was passed on to her closest students, and has survived, grossly coarsened, to the present day.[3]

It is apparent that Rudolf Steiner found the oriental occultism of the Viennese disciples of Madame Blavatsky little to his taste. For him it seemed lacking in that contact with the spiritual realities which he instinctively felt must underlie the world of matter. It was not that Eckstein and those associated with him were lacking in intelligence and sophistication. It was that with them he had not sensed himself in the presence of those who had refreshed themselves with the living waters of the supersensual life. Such refreshment, he was sure, was obtainable, for he had observed its effects upon an illiterate herbalist whom he had first met in the course of a suburban railway journey.

The man in question, a factory worker of peasant background, who in his spare time gathered herbs and practised what would today be called alternative medicine, was named Felix Kogutzki. His herbal knowledge seems to have been instinctive rather than traditional – that is to say he selected the appropriate herbal remedy for a particular patient on the basis of what he felt rather than what he knew. This intuitive approach, today a feature of at least some anthroposophical medical practice, impressed Steiner, who felt that he was in the presence of a natural mystic, a man who was (as he put it) 'the mouthpiece for a spiritual content from hidden worlds', the bringer of 'an instinctive knowledge from the past'.

Without underestimating the effect upon Steiner of his encounters with Kogutzki, these contacts were in some ways less important for the development of Steiner's 'spiritual science' than was his exposure to the writings of Franz von Hartmann; it would not be going too far to say that it was Steiner's reaction against Hartmann's pessimistic philosophy which led him first to formulate that 'philosophy of freedom' which is the foundation stone of the theory which underlies the practical techniques of anthroposophical education, art, agriculture and medicine.

In his own day von Hartmann was sometimes referred to as 'the philosopher of the Unconscious'. This was apt enough, for von Hartmann believed that 'the motor of evolution' – to use a phrase coined by one of his disciples – was a deep unconscious will to life, an instinctive force which was in every way the antithesis of intellect and rational thought. Intellect, which von Hartmann sometimes referred to as 'daylight consciousness', has caused man to be aware of his instincts and, even worse, of the utter pointlessness of the evolutionary process of which they are the driving force. There was, said von Hartmann, no rational purpose to life; everything was, in the most absolute sense, hopeless, all mankind's vaunted achievements were no more than exercises in futility.

Steiner was so disturbed by von Hartmann's gloom and doom that he travelled to the latter's Berlin home with the intention of raising various objections to the philosopher's all-embracing pessimism.[4] Von Hartmann, mistaking Steiner for an enthusiastic but muddled disciple, replied brusquely to his questions and, according to Steiner's own account, 'did not inwardly *listen* to what was said'. Steiner was particularly shocked by von Hartmann's statement that the term 'mental pictures', as applied to the images present in consciousness, necessarily implies that these 'pictures' are, by definition, unreal. 'I felt inwardly chilled', wrote Steiner, 'by the use of word-definition as the point of departure for a philosophy of life.'

Steiner's *Philosophy of Freedom* (1894) was his closely reasoned response to von Hartmann's materialism, denial of free will and assertion of cosmic futility. Materialism, asserted Steiner, is inherently incapable of satisfactorily explaining existence. For any such explanation 'must begin with the formation of *thoughts* about the phenomena of the world. Materialism thus begins with the *thought* of matter or material processes. In doing so it is immediately confronted by two different sets of facts: the world of matter itself and the thoughts about it.' In other words, spiritual activity, of which the thought of a materialist philosopher is a particular manifestation, arises out of freedom. In his incomplete autobiography Steiner summed up his purpose in writing the *Philosophy of Freedom*:

I tried to show . . . that nothing *unknowable* lies behind the sense-world, but that *within* it is the spiritual world. And I tried to show that man's idea-world has its existence within the spiritual world. Therefore the true reality of the sense-world remains hidden from human consciousness *only* for *as long as* man is merely engaged in sense perception.

In essence this paragraph sums up the basis of the spiritual science which Steiner was to formulate in the years 1900–1925.

Four years before the publication of the *Philosophy of Freedom* Rudolf Steiner's reputation as a Goethe scholar had led to his being offered a post at the Goethe Archive in Weimar. He had accepted with alacrity; quite apart from the fact that his salary from the Archive would be a more reliable source of income than that earned by tutoring and literary work, the job gave him that academic respectability which, like most German-speaking scholars of his time, he considered desirable. In the following year the seal, so to speak, was put on his academic reputation when the University of Rostock accepted his thesis on a theory of cognition and conferred a doctorate upon him.

Steiner was not as happy at Weimar as might have been expected. He found the intellectual atmosphere of the Archive cloyingly pedantic, and, in 1897, he threw up his job and moved to Berlin, where he earned a sparse living by writing and lecturing to such bodies as the Workers' Circle, a Social Democratic – which at that date meant Marxist – educational association. Steiner was not, of course, a Marxist, and there is no doubt that he had always rejected Marx and Engels's materialist interpretation of history which he had first encountered in the Vienna of the 1880s. He wrote:

It was painful for me to hear it said that in human history it is the material-economic factors that are decisive for man's evolution, while the spiritual is only the superstructure erected on this 'truly real' foundation. I knew that the spirit is a reality. For me to accept what the theorizing socialists maintained would have meant closing my eyes to the facts.

It is interesting to note that in spite of his rejection of historical materialism the proletarian students of the Workers' Circle found Steiner's lectures acceptable. Clearly he had mastered the technique of expressing the content of his thought in a form which a particular audience would find palatable; it would seem that Steiner was able to sugar the pill of philosophical idealism with a coating of Marxist dialectical materialism.

At some time in the summer of 1900 a member of the Berlin Lodge of the Theosophical Society read a curious article by Steiner on the hidden significance of Goethe's fairy tale *The Green Serpent and the Beautiful Lily* and arranged that he should be asked to give the lodge a lecture on the same subject. The lecture, in which Steiner gave a somewhat strained esoteric interpretation of Goethe's story, was given towards the end of September; it met with approval and was succeeded by a series of lectures on mystics, mysticism and, in the winter of 1901–2, 'Christianity as Mystical Fact'.

None of these lectures seems to have shown any great originality of thought – indeed, Steiner's ideas on the 'Mystical Fact' of Christianity seem to have been very largely derived from the writings of the French occultist Edouard Schuré – but the members of the Berlin Lodge felt, and felt rightly, that their content was subtly different from the usual run of Theosophical propaganda, that here was a change of emphasis.

Some of Steiner's audience found this disturbing, sensing the presence of 'Theosophical heresy', and one lodge member pointed out to Steiner that his teachings differed from those of Annie Besant, the dominant figure in the Theosophical

Society since the death of Madame Blavatsky and the eclipse of W. Q. Judge. 'Is that the case?' murmured Steiner politely, and carried on, as before, emphasizing the European elements in the world's mystical traditions. Such critics, however, were in a minority. Most of the members of the Berlin Lodge found Steiner's approach to their taste and, more important, came to the conclusion that it resulted from direct experience of spiritual realities.

By the summer of 1902 this attitude was so general amongst German-speaking Theosophists that the German Section of the society was reorganized with Steiner as its general secretary. Within a few years Steiner's influence began to extend beyond the German-speaking world, largely as the result of his close friendship with Marie von Sivers (1867–1948), a Baltic German – that is to say, a German-speaking subject of the Russian Empire – who was later to become his wife.

Marie von Sivers, an actress, dancer and student of occult literature, had first met Steiner at one of his early lectures to the Berlin Theosophists and there is good reason to think that it was she who induced him to throw in his lot with what was, at that time, a small and largely ineffectual movement. Amongst her acquaintances and friends in the Russian expatriate community in Berlin were a number of Russian writers, painters and other intellectuals with a vague interest in occultism in general and Theosophy in particular and, in 1905, she arranged for Steiner to give a series of lectures to these exiles.

The lectures, which were given in the informal surroundings of Marie von Sivers's apartment, were greeted with some enthusiasm, and it was planned that Steiner should visit Russia in the summer of the following year in order to acquaint himself with the Theosophical movement in that country and, of course, to deliver further lectures. This plan had to be abandoned because of the chaotic political and social upheavals which resulted from the abortive Russian Revolution of 1905–6 and the lectures were instead delivered in Paris, at that time the Western capital of the Russian intellectual emigration.

Steiner's choice of dates for the delivery of his 'Russian'

lectures was a fortunate one, coinciding as it did with the world conference of the Theosophical Society, also being held in Paris. His audience included a number of distinguished avant-garde Russian intellectuals, amongst them the poetess Zenaida Hippius and the Symbolist novelist Dmitri Merezhkovsky, and his ideas and the way in which he expressed them were well received. Steiner, in short, enjoyed a minor triumph over Annie Besant and the official leadership of the Theosophical Society, for his Parisian lecture cycle received rather more attention than did the proceedings of the official gathering to which he was, of course, a delegate. To all intents and purposes Steiner had held a rival, unofficial, world Theosophical conference and, in the process of doing so, had created an awareness of himself as a serious claimant to Theosophical leadership, a formidable rival to Annie Besant and those close to her. It was clear to those Theosophists with foresight that, sooner or later, their society would split in two; its national sections and individual members would have to choose between Europe and Asia, between Rudolf Steiner and Annie Besant.

The choice would not be between rival personalities but between ideologies, between the Christ-centred Theosophy of Steiner with its concern for that European esoteric tradition which has as its symbols the rose and the cross and the increasingly eccentric pseudo-oriental teachings of the official leadership, men and women whose beliefs were fairly summed up by Friedrich Rittelmeyer as being 'a mixture of ancient tradition and subjective emotionalism'.

For the next few years there was an uneasy relationship, marked by a guarded hostility, between Rudolf Steiner and the world leadership of the Theosophical Society. The former began to gain influence amongst the Theosophists of Holland, France and Russia, while even in England, where Annie Besant had a surprisingly large personal following, Steiner's 'Rosicrucian Theosophy' had its adherents.

Not surprisingly, Annie Besant became worried and there is some evidence that she and her advisers began to encourage the formation of anti-Steiner groupings within the German movement. One of those most prominent in the activities of such groups was Hugo Vollrath (1877–circa 1942), a man who had ceased his formal education before he had finished his university studies but, none the less, fraudulently styled himself Herr Doktor Vollrath until the summer of 1914.⁵

In 1907 Vollrath participated in the establishment of a small occult publishing house situated in Leipzig. This city had an active Theosophical group, the members of which, believing that Vollrath was possessed of some literary expertise, appointed him as their librarian. Almost immediately Vollrath abused his position, using the facilities provided by the Leipzig group to announce the formation of a Literary Society of the German Section of the Theosophical Society, with himself as its *de facto* head under a board of 'Honorary Patrons' whose names were used without their permission or even knowledge; it would seem that Vollrath's 'Literary Society' was little more than an attempt, first, to present commercial publishing activities as being under official Theosophical patronage, and, secondly, to set up an alternative, anti-Steiner centre.

The Leipzig Theosophists felt that they were being used for Vollrath's personal purposes and made complaints to Steiner in his official capacity as general secretary of the German Section. Steiner, not surprisingly, was sympathetic to the attitude of the Leipzig group and at the conference of the German Theosophists which took place in October 1908 formally announced Vollrath's expulsion from the movement.

Vollrath, who had some support amongst the old guard of German Theosophy, men and women who had known and admired Madame Blavatsky, was totally unrepentant and appealed to Annie Besant and the world leadership, who gave him at least partial support. Rudolf Steiner, it was decided, had acted within his powers when he had expelled Vollrath from the German Section; but this expulsion did not, so it was held, in any way affect Vollrath's relationship with the international Theosophical Society, of which he remained a member in good standing. Not long after this curious judgement, as if to emphasise her support for Vollrath, Annie Besant appointed the bogus Herr Doktor as German representative of that eccentric body the Order of the Star of the East. The order in question had been founded

in 1911, its function being to announce a forthcoming manifestation of the 'World Teacher' – in other words, a new
incarnation of Christ. According to Annie Besant, this event
was imminent. In the near future the World Teacher would
take over the body of Jiddu Krishnamurti, a young Indian
boy who was the son of a minor employee at the society's
headquarters in Madras.[6]

The teachings associated with the Order of the Star were
deeply repellent to Steiner and those who, like him, had come
to believe that the incarnation of Christ was a unique and
supremely important event in world history; so far as the
majority of German Theosophists were concerned, the
propaganda emanating from the order was no more than
a grotesque blasphemy, and membership of the order was
declared incompatible with membership of the German
Section. Nothing could have been more calculated to
infuriate Mrs Besant and her satraps on the general council
of the Theosophical Society. Steiner's German Section was
suspended from membership of the international organization and a rival German Section – to which, in fact, only
fourteen lodges out of a total of sixty-nine adhered – was
set up. In February 1913 the split was made apparent to all
by Steiner's society changing its name to the Anthroposophical Society. The change of name was no mere formality;
there is no doubt that Steiner was right to distinguish
between the Theosophy of the devotees of Krishnamurti and
the very different Rosicrucian Theosophy which he had
developed – or perhaps encountered as the result of
employing supersensual modes of perception – over the
preceding years.[7]

Steiner was now the chief of a small but growing international movement which needed a world headquarters.
Originally it was planned that this should be in Germany,
either at Munich or Stuttgart, but eventually a hill on the
outskirts of Dornach, Switzerland, became the chosen site
and, in September 1913, the foundation stone of the
building, known as the Goetheanum, was laid.

By the outbreak of war in August 1914 the main structure
of the Goetheanum, which was built almost entirely of
timber (according to some reports of the same seven varieties

of wood as those supposedly used by such master violin makers as Stradivarius), was largely complete. It seemed to some to be a triumphant affirmation of the forces of light and spirituality, a contrast to the darkness and death of wartorn Europe, and throughout the years of war men and women of all nationalities continued to work together harmoniously at Dornach, but not without increasing opposition from forces hostile to anthroposophy.

Such hostility came from three main sources: representatives of orthodox Protestantism, who looked upon Steiner as some sort of neo-Gnostic and felt his Christocentric occultism to be a dangerous heresy; extreme nationalist politicians, ideological forerunners of Nazism, who regarded the entire Anthroposophical Society as no more than a front for a Jewish-Marxist conspiracy to take over the world; and students of mysticism, who claimed that anthroposophy was tainted with black magic.

The latter grouping was responsible for spreading some very odd rumours. It was said, for example, that Rudolf Steiner had murdered his first wife by means of 'astral strangulation', that he habitually practised 'sex magic', and that he had been responsible for a young schoolmistress giving birth to an 'astral child'. The oddest accusations of all were made by a certain Herr Krieger, who issued a newsletter in which he asserted that Steiner and other anthroposophists were guilty of astral vampirism and had stolen his soul. Krieger even went to the length of conducting an unsuccessful legal case against Steiner; many years after it had begun the farce ended in tragedy when, in 1929, Krieger murdered Dr Carl Unger, whom he believed to have been Rudolf Steiner's accomplice in the act of spiritual theft.

It was also asserted that the spiritual exercises advocated by Steiner were mentally and physically dangerous, and in 1917 the magazine *Psychische Studien* carried a report that the artist Erich Bamler had become suicidally depressed as a result of their use, while 'Dr Kobylinsky of Berlin' – who was probably identical with the Russian poet Kobylinsky-Ellis – denounced anthroposophy as 'kabalistic magic with its always attendant cynicism, avarice and sex magic' and categorically stated that his own experiments with Steiner's exercises had resulted in heart disease.

Kobylinsky's accusations of sex magic were to prove a recurring feature of anti-Steiner polemics[8] and are still sometimes repeated at the present day. They arose out of Steiner's brief involvement with what is sometimes called 'esoteric masonry' and his consequent leadership of a small secret society called Mysteria Mystica Aeterna.

The origins of this society are to be found in the activities of a certain John Yarker, a Victorian Freemason, a respectable resident of Manchester, who collected masonic rites, dignities and obscure charters as another man might collect coins or postage stamps. Amongst the many masonic rites of which Yarker obtained leadership, largely because no one else was in any way interested in them, was the Rite of Memphis and Misraim, which was of obscure and uncertain origin, although it may have had links with the occult masonry of the eighteenth century. In his later years Yarker lived in great poverty and his tiny income was almost entirely derived from the fees he received in return for 'charters' empowering their recipients to establish working lodges of Memphis and Misraim.

In 1902 Yarker issued a charter of this sort to three German occultists, Theodor Reuss, Joshua Klein and Franz Hartmann, the old disciple of Madame Blavatsky. Reuss was undoubtedly the dominant figure in the partnership and seems to have operated the grandiloquently entitled Berlin Lodge of Memphis and Misraim with no other end in view than the extraction of large fees from the gullible. In 1904 a society usually referred to as the OTO became amalgamated or associated with Reuss's Grand Lodge. The OTO was the Ordens Tempel der Ostens, the Order of Oriental Templars, which undoubtedly taught a variety of sexual magic – that is to say, supposedly spiritual exercises involving physical sexuality which were analogous to, perhaps even derived from, the left-handed Tantra of Bengal.[9] Tantra is a system of physical, mental and spiritual disciplines incorporating meditation, yoga and varieties of sacramental worship involving polarity concepts. In left-handed Tantra physical sexuality, in effect the orgasm as a sacrament, is employed by devotees of the cult. The phrase 'left-handed' refers to the fact that in the preliminary stages the female devotee sits on her partner's left side.

How Steiner was first brought into contact with this body is uncertain, but there is no doubt that at some time prior to the spring of 1906 he acquired from it a charter to operate, under the name Mysteria Mystica Aeterna, a 'Chapter and Grand Council' of the rite. There is no reason to doubt the purity of Steiner's motives in obtaining his charter. In his own words, he 'never thought of working in the spirit of such a society. . . . I took nothing . . . from this society except the merely formal authorisation, in historic succession, to direct a symbolic-cultural activity.' It was an unwise move, however, and while one can be confident that Steiner never practised sexual magic one can understand how it was that he came to be accused of doing so.[10]

There seems to be little substance to the accusations that the use of Steiner's exercises, such as those recommended in *Knowledge of the Higher Worlds and Its Attainment*, has led to physical or mental illness. This is not to say that some of those who have used these exercises have not become neurotic or even psychotic. But it is impossible to reasonably argue 'after this, therefore on account of this' in relation to such neuroses and psychoses; like all movements concerned with the things of the spirit, from the Roman Catholic Church to Zen Buddhism, anthroposophy has attracted its quota of oddballs and madmen. From my own limited experience I think it likely that the Anthroposophical Society has attracted rather a smaller proportion of such disturbed individuals than has been attracted by some other esoteric and quasi-esoteric organizations.

Extreme nationalist political opposition to Rudolf Steiner seems to have had its origins in his close relationship with General von Moltke, Chief of the German General Staff at the outbreak of war in August 1914. Both von Moltke and his wife were enthusiastic advocates of Steiner's ideas, the former once having been reported as saying that 'Steiner's Theosophy is the only great philosophy that has no gaps.' At the outbreak of war von Moltke seems to have been extremely indecisive, unable to make up his mind whether or not to apply in their entirety contingency plans drawn up by the General Staff many years before and intended to deliver a decisive blow against France. The choice von Moltke had to make was by no means such an easy one as his critics have sometimes maintained; there was no doubt that if the plans were successfully executed France would be defeated in a matter of weeks, but, on the other hand, if they failed Germany herself could be invaded and a victorious French army might parade through Berlin.

The choice von Moltke made was unfortunate. He applied the plan only partially, the German advance was halted, and four years of bloody trench warfare followed. The ultra-nationalists, unable to accept that Germany was not invincible, blamed Rudolf Steiner for what had happened. Either, they said, Steiner had given the General wrong advice or, alternatively, von Moltke was so dependent upon Steiner that he had been unable to make a decision until he had consulted him. In reality there is no evidence at all that Steiner's advice, or failure to give advice, affected von Moltke's decision in any way whatsoever. Nevertheless, from September 1914 onwards Steiner and the Anthroposophical Society were regarded with considerable and steadily increasing suspicion by the lunatic fringe of German nationalism.

Steiner made matters worse by deciding, towards the end of the war, that the time was ripe for the propagation of his own political and social theories, which seem to have evolved from the system of 'synarchy' advocated by the French occultist Saint-Yves d'Alveydre (1842–1909) and popularized by the writer 'Papus' (Dr Gerard Encausse) in such books as *What is Occultism?* (Rider, 1913). The basis of synarchy, which Saint-Yves said meant 'totalism', was the application of a triune concept of the human organism to human society. The cephalic, rhythmic and metabolic-limb systems of the human body were to have their sociological counterparts in the spiritual, legislative and economic life of each nation.

Between the spring of 1917 and that of 1919 Steiner elaborated and refined his version of synarchy, which he called 'the Threefold Commonwealth', and in April of the latter year he published a book of the same title. It sold extremely well and a quasi-political organization, the Union for the Threefold Social Order, was established.

Synarchy, even with Steiner's modifications, did not appeal to either the left or the right. The Marxists regarded it as an idealistic attempt to divert the working class from its historic task of smashing the bourgeois state machine and establishing a dictatorship of the proletariat, while the nationalist parties, including the groups which were to coalesce into the Nazi Party, saw it as an expression of 'parlour Bolshevism' and 'Jewish internationalism'. The attacks made upon Steiner by Dietrich Eckart, a proto-Nazi who exerted a strong influence on the political development of Adolf Hitler, were particularly virulent. Steiner, he said, was a totally untrustworthy Galician Jew, a megalomaniac whose driving force was his greed for money, a practitioner of sexual magic who was the agent of a Jewish-Masonic-Bolshevik conspiracy.

Such nationalist opposition to Steiner steadily increased. In 1922 he was physically attacked by young Nazis; it became almost impossible for him to deliver a public lecture in Germany without being subjected to constant heckling; and, on the last night of the year, the Goetheanum was almost entirely destroyed by fire. This last may have been accidental, but there were strong suspicions, never allayed, that arson had been involved. Some suspected that the supposed fire raisers had been German nationalists, perhaps young Nazis, from Bavaria; others that they had been Swiss, fanatical Protestants, whose feelings had been aroused by the opposition of the local pastors. One such cleric received a postcard from an angry anthroposophist which bore the words: 'Who are the arsonists?' The pastor, reasonably enough, replied that it would perhaps be best to ask Dr Steiner that question 'as it is he who is supposed to have clairvoyant powers'.

The building of a new Goetheanum began immediately. Concrete, not timber, was the material used in the second construction which, like the first, was designed by Steiner himself. He also planned its decor, which was no mere piece of interior design but a conscious attempt to express spiritual realities through the use of clay, stone, wood and glass.

Steiner died in March 1925; the Goetheanum abides, and is now the centre of a worldwide movement.

Over the quarter of a century or so which preceded the destruction of the first Goetheanum Rudolf Steiner wrote several books and delivered approximately six thousand lectures. These latter were concerned with the spiritual dimensions of an incredible variety of subjects, from beekeeping to architecture, from dancing to the everyday life of legendary drowned Atlantis, but one of the common threads which links them all is an underlying belief in the value of *conscious* reasoning based upon normal and super-normal modes of perception. I have emphasized the word 'conscious' because it is apparent that Rudolf Steiner considered unacceptable the very idea of the existence of an impenetrable Unconscious, inaccessible to both self-obser-vation and rational thought processes, the domain of the mindless, instinctive drives of Franz von Hartmann and his disciples. While he seems to have accepted that human beings *can* be controlled by unconscious desires, drives and processes, he felt that there is no necessity for them to be thus controlled. For Steiner nothing needs to remain below the level of consciousness. The Unconscious can become conscious and mankind is capable of perceiving the cosmic totality in all its aspects through the use of Imagination, Inspiration and Intuition. These words have been capitalized because, when used within the context of Steiner's anthro-posophy, they are endowed with particular meanings which differ from those of colloquial English usage. For students of the teachings of Rudolf Steiner Imagination, Inspiration and Intuition refer to, respectively, etheric, astral and spiri-tual modes of perception. To understand what is meant by this latter phrase, essential if the theoretical bases of anthroposophical medicine are to be comprehended, it is important to acquire at least an outline knowledge of the system expounded by Steiner during the years in which he built up the anthroposophical movement. It is a system which concerns both 'the kingdoms of nature and the nature of Man'.

2

The Kingdoms of Nature and the Nature of Man

The natural philosophers of old looked upon mankind as being, quite literally, the Lord of Creation, a triple monarch ruling over the animal, vegetable and mineral kingdoms. There is some blurring at the edges between the borders of these kingdoms. Is a virus a complex chemical or is it endowed with life? Is a hydra an animal or a plant? None the less, the classification of the contents of our world into these three divisions is still a useful one and, if Rudolf Steiner's teachings are accepted, it does accurately represent underlying realities.

'Underlying' is a key word for understanding the teachings of Rudolf Steiner in general and those which have resulted in the emergence of anthroposophical medicine in particular. For the anthroposophist regards the world of animate and inanimate matter perceived by the five senses as being only one aspect of reality. Underlying that world of matter are, so it is believed, other worlds and other modes of being. Even dense matter is held to have locked within it, as though in some temporal deep freeze, the imprints of the processes which formed its constituent parts; as will be explained in chapter 3, anthroposophical pharmacists endeavour to release these locked-in processes, thus making them available for therapeutic purposes, by techniques referred to as dynamization or potentization. Furthermore, the separate components of the world of matter continuously give rise to subtle force flows, incapable of laboratory measurement or perception through the normal channels of the senses, which interconnect with, and have affinities for, other seemingly discrete physical entities – there is, for example, such an interconnection between the sun and the physical structure of the human heart.

The existence of three 'worlds', that is, of three modes of existence (and consciousness) apart from that of inanimate matter, is a fundamental premise of anthroposophy and the system of holistic therapeutics which has been derived from it. They are, in ascending order of their 'separation' from physical manifestation, the etheric, the astral and the spiritual.

In some ways the first two of these names are unfortunate. 'Etheric' is somewhat suggestive of the hypothetical and now abandoned concept of an invisible interplanetary continuum, called 'ether', through which travel light and electromagnetic waves, while 'astral' is a word which has been so overused by fraudulent mediums and self-deceiving prophets of dubious spirituality that it has acquired an almost pejorative meaning. It is worth saying, then, that, while the word 'etheric' has the same root as that from which was derived the 'ether' of pre-Einsteinian physics, the words do not express identical concepts. The 'etheric forces' of anthroposophy are in no way connected with the transmission of electricity, magnetism, light or gravitational forces through space; they are, so Rudolf Steiner taught his pupils, the formative forces which underlie and shape all animate matter, thus ensuring, for example, that a buttercup has the form appropriate to a buttercup, not that of an oak tree or a cabbage. Etheric forces determine particular physical forms, and it is possible to refer to the physical/etheric complex of a plant, an animal or a human organism and, likewise, to refer to the 'etheric bodies' of all these forms of life.

Etheric forces as such cannot be directly perceived as sense impressions or measured by normal laboratory techniques. Many anthroposophical physicians believe, however, that it is possible to obtain an image of the *effects* of etheric forces by a technique known as sensitive crystallization. This technique, originally devised by the late Ehrenfried Pfeiffer, involves adding a few drops of liquid from plant or animal material (blood or sap, for example) to a chemical solution, usually copper chloride, and letting it crystallize. The crystalline patterns which result, and no two of which ever seem to be absolutely identical, present an image, so it is averred, of the etheric forces at work in the plant, animal or human being from which the liquid extract was taken. The interpretation of these images is an art not a science, and requires skill, experience and a certain indefinable flair. Those experienced in the use of this technique claim that, when applied to human blood, it is an invaluable aid to the diagnosis of pathological conditions at a preclinical stage, that is, before any overt symptoms have become apparent.

The word 'astral' simply means 'sidereal', 'starry'; the phrase 'astral body' was first coined by Paracelsus, who used it to mean the non-physical vehicle of consciousness through which the stars — in this context meaning subtle cosmic influences — interact with human and animal organisms. It is in very much this same sense that Steiner used the phrase: astral bodies, which are not possessed by plants, supposedly underlie the etheric bodies of animals and men in very much the same way in which etheric forces are believed to underlie, form and pattern their physical bodies.

The components of the mineral kingdom, then, have only a physical form or body; they can in geometrical terms be considered analogous to a straight line, which exists in only one dimension. Plants, the components of the vegetable kingdom, have both physical and etheric bodies; they are analogous to squares, triangles and other two-dimensional figures. Animals have all three dimensions and are analogous to solid figures such as cubes and spheres — that is, they have physical, etheric and astral bodies. Human beings also have these three bodies but they are extended into a mysterious fourth dimension of spirituality, for at the core of each individual man or woman is the immortal spirit, the central 'I', usually referred to by anthroposophists as the 'Ego'.

Steiner asserted that, enclosed within the Ego, are the seeds of higher stages of development. He said:

The Ego . . . encloses and develops within it the seeds of higher stages. . . . Man consists of a physical body, an etheric body, an astral body, and the Ego, the real inner Life; and within this inner Life are the rudiments of three more advanced stages of development. . . . These three are Spirit self [the transmuted astral body], Life spirit [the transmuted etheric body], and Spirit man [the transmuted physical body]; the Spirit self as distinguished from the bodily self, the Life spirit, and the true Spirit man, a distant ideal to the contemporary man . . . but fated to reach perfection in the far off future.

We have seven colours in the rainbow, seven tones in the scale . . . and seven grades in the scale of the human being, divided into four lower and three higher grades . . . this higher triad achieves a physiognomical expression in the lower quaternary.[1]

It is this last-mentioned lower quaternary and the interactions between its components that are of particular relevance to anthroposophical medicine.

An easy way to visualize these components – physical, etheric, astral and spiritual – and the relationships between them is to think of the physical body as permeated by the etheric body, which is itself permeated by the astral body, which in its turn is permeated by the Ego. The carrying out of such image making, which was suggested by Steiner himself, is helpful if one wishes to construct some sort of pictorial model of the quaternary as a whole. It must always be remembered, however, that such a model cannot, by definition, be more than an approximation to reality, and that the Ego and the astral body enjoy an existence which is beyond the narrow limits of three-dimensional space – they are in no sense to be understood as shadowy, attenuated images of the physical body.

It is to the etheric, astral and spiritual worlds and modes of consciousness that pertain the higher modes of perception, referred to in the preceding chapter, which Steiner termed Imagination, Inspiration and Intuition.

Speaking of mankind's relationship to the etheric world Steiner asserted that the

etheric body . . . far from being an invented hypothesis is as distinctly visible to the developed spiritual senses of the esotericist as are externally perceptible colours to physical sight. This etheric body can actually be seen by the clairvoyant. It is the principle which calls inorganic matter into life . . . weaving them [inorganic molecules] into the warp and weft of life's garment. Do not imagine that this body is to the esotericist merely something which he adds in thought to the inanimate. . . .

Now man is in a state of evolution, and for this reason anthroposophy says: 'If you remain as you are you will not see the etheric body . . . but if you develop and acquire the necessary faculties for the cognition of spiritual things you will no longer speak of the "boundaries of knowledge", for these exist only so long as man has not developed his inner senses.'

The higher mode of perception, which is particularly concerned with direct experience of the etheric formative forces, is what Steiner referred to as Imagination, so called because when this faculty is employed consciousness is filled with 'living pictures' in comparison to which the pictorial images of everyday consciousness are 'mere shadows of thought'. Steiner insisted that the faculty of Imagination confers the ability actually to *see* – that is, to perceive spiritually – the etheric realities which are present in man, animals and plants. He also argued that the faculty of etheric vision is qualitatively, not quantitatively, different from ordinary processes of thought and sense perception, an extension of the human cognitive faculties which enables the experience of an extended reality.

The Imaginative faculty is exercised when consciousness has been emptied of physically pictorial impressions and filled with etherically pictorial impressions. When these also have been removed from the consciousness of an individual human being that individual reaches a state of voidness in which he or she is still conscious, fully awake and aware, *but the awareness is devoid of content*. Into that voidness pour astral impressions; knowledge by Inspiration has been achieved, the realities of the astral world are perceived in their entirety.

The next stage is the achievement of Intuitive knowledge. This faculty of Intuition is an essentially human attribute, raising mankind to a level above that of the animal kingdom, for of all the animate beings which share our planet only men and women are, in the fullest sense, spirit beings, possessed of what Steiner termed the Ego. The man or woman who has attained to Intuition, said Steiner, has brought the spiritual to full consciousness and has been born to a new life in which he or she is a spirit being dwelling amidst other spirit beings.

Rudolf Steiner devised a system of what might be termed spiritual athletic training, that is, graduated exercises designed to develop higher modes of perception, which he claimed could be used in order to attain direct knowledge of underlying realities through the employment of Imagination, Inspiration and Intuition. Even the briefest description of these excercises lies outside the scope of this book. It suffices to say that it is claimed by some who have used them that they have attained, in some measure at least, the exercise of those higher modes of perception through which Steiner claimed to have acquired the knowledge which provides the theoretical underpinnings of anthroposophical medical practice. This knowledge is generally concerned with the functions of the spiritual, astral, etheric and physical aspects of the human totality, with the interactions of these component aspects, and with the etheric formative forces as they are at work in plant, animal and man.

Steiner taught that there is a particular relationship between each component of the human quaternary and one of the four elements of the ancients, that is to say, Earth, Air, Fire and Water. The Ego, he said, relates to the element of Fire and the warmth associated with it, the astral body relates to the element of Air, the etheric to Water, and the physical to Earth. This terminology is sometimes productive of difficulties and has caused some critics to accuse Steiner of holding antiquated and mistaken concepts, ideas which have been abandoned by all sensible men for over three centuries. Such criticism shows, I think, a lack of awareness of Steiner's way of expressing his teachings. When he used the word 'element' in relation to, say, 'Water' he was not using that word in the same sense that it is used by someone making some such statement as 'nitrogen is an element'. Nor, when he referred to 'Water' and 'Fire', did he mean the water with which a kettle is filled and the fire which heats that kettle. What he was doing, I feel sure, was what many mystics have tried, and usually failed, to do – to communicate the

nature of spiritual realities in language which can be comprehended by those who have had no direct experience of such
realities. It is impossible to communicate the precise nature
of what is experienced when using the visual faculty to
someone who has been blind from birth. Usually the best
one can do is to use some sort of analogy – to say, for
example, that the difference between two colours resembles
the difference between two musical notes.

The mystic has the same difficulty when he or she endeavours to explain his or her perceptions to those who have
never experienced altered states of consciousness. All that
can be done is to use analogies similiar to those in which
colours are compared to musical notes; an endeavour is made
to describe what is *beyond* the world of sense impressions
in terms comprehensible to those who have had no experience of worlds other than those capable of perception by the
senses.

It is probable that Steiner adopted his seemingly antiquated
terminology of the four elements for very similar reasons.
That which he perceived through the attainment of higher
modes of perception and consciousness was inherently
incapable of being explained in its entirety through the use
of human language, for language has evolved as a method
of communicating the content of sense impressions (and
thoughts concerning, or deriving from, that content) from
one human being to another. I believe that Steiner used the
words 'Water' and 'Air' in relation to, respectively, the astral
and etheric worlds because the water we drink and the air
we breathe have qualities which dimly shadow forth and
are, in a sense, reflective qualities which are particularly
associated with the astral and etheric realities of which he
had direct apprehension and comprehension.

The same is, I suspect, true of many other terms used
by Rudolf Steiner and still employed in anthroposophical
medicine: for example, the words 'salt', 'sulphur' and
'mercury' are sometimes used by anthroposophical pharmacists and physicians in a sense different from that in which
they are used in ordinary language, reference being made,
for example, to 'the mercury' of a plant substance, which
does not, in fact, contain any trace of the chemical element

of that name; or, perhaps even more confusingly, certain aspects of the functioning of the human body being described as pertaining to its 'salt pole' or its 'sulphur pole'. Steiner seems to have derived the usage of these terms from the writings of Paracelsus and his followers, the spagyric – that is, alchemical – physicians. There is nothing surprising in such a derivation, for Steiner was well acquainted with the writings of those physicians of his own time who were students of esoteric subjects, men such as Dr Gerard Encausse (Papus) and Dr Franz Hartmann, mentioned above, both of whom had published books on occult medicine which were largely based on Paracelsian concepts.

The exact nature of the concepts which Rudolf Steiner wished to express by his Paracelsian usage of the words 'salt', 'sulphur' and 'mercury' is not easy to convey. There is a sense in which they are subtler, less intense versions of the elements of, respectively, Earth, Fire and Water. Possibly they are best described as principles, cosmic processes which are embodied in animate and inanimate matter. In this case it is legitimate to think of the mercury in our thermometers, the sulphur which is contained in gunpowder and the salt we put on our potatoes as material substances which 'personify' these cosmic processes of the three Paracelsian principles.

At around the turn of the last century Dr Encausse as Papus wrote extensively on the subject of occult medicine, classifying the functions of the human organism in accord-ance with the Paracelsian principles. He grouped these func-tions into three categories, which he called 'eating', 'living' and 'thinking'. 'Eating', by which word Papus seems to have intended to describe the metabolic processes as a whole, was equated with the sulphur of Paracelsus; 'living', a word used to indicate the pulmonary and circulatory processes, was ascribed to mercury; and 'thinking', which included all cerebral and nerve activity, was equated with salt.

A very similar triune division of the human organism and its functions was taught by Steiner and is today adhered to by practitioners of anthroposophical medicine. The first of these divisions is called the 'cephalic pole', centred on the head but extending throughout the entire body as the nerve-sense system. The cephalic or upper pole is sometimes referred to as the 'salt pole', which seems to indicate its equivalence to the 'thinking' category. The lower pole, equated by Rudolf Steiner with sulphur and frequently referred to as the 'pole of metabolism' or 'limb-metabolism' – locomotion is regarded, reasonably enough, as an extension and outcome of the metabolic process – seems to be more or less the same as the system to which Papus crudely referred to as 'eating'. The two poles, cephalic and metabolic, Paracelsian salt and sulphur, are harmonized in their function by the mercurial principle, the rhythmic system centred on the thorax and concerned with such functions as breathing and the circulation of the blood.

The two poles and the rhythmic system which is believed to mediate between them must not be thought of as confined to one area of the body, but operating throughout it. Thus the pulmonary-circulatory processes of the rhythm system operate in the head, which is the centre of the nerve-sense system, which pertains to the cephalic pole. Similarly the nerve-sense system extends into such components of the metabolic-limb system as the stomach and the feet, while that system itself extends into areas of the body which pertain more particularly to the nerve-sense and rhythmic systems.

The cephalic pole, taught Rudolf Steiner, is concerned with thought, consciousness and the perceptions of the senses – light, sound, smell and so on. It is in a sense the centripetal element in the human biosystem, that which draws inward and absorbs from outside the system. In contrast the metabolic, or motor-digestive, pole is centrifugal in its tendencies, directly influencing the outside world through the actions of the will. The two opposing tendencies are, in the healthy organism, kept in exact and harmonious balance with one another by the rhythmic system, which unites thought with the will through which the individual acts upon his environment.

In the metabolic-limb system the etheric formative forces, the forces which transform inert matter into living tissue, are extremely active, with the reproductive organs, integral parts of that system, emphasizing the 'living' nature of motor-digestive processes.

In the nerve-sense system there is no such intense etheric

activity expressing itself in cellular renewal and multiplication. On the contrary, it is the processes which culminate in stasis and, eventually, physical death which are dominant – brain and nerve cells are incapable of renewal and replacement. This means, say students of anthroposophical medicine, that the etheric forces at work in the nerve-sense system, instead of being transmuted into physical forms – cells – are transmuted into thought, memory and the power of associating ideas into chainlike logical structures. This means that at the cephalic pole there is a much less close link between the etheric and physical bodies than that which obtains at the motor-digestive pole, and, conversely, that there is a closer linkage between the etheric and astral bodies at the cephalic pole than at the metabolic, motor-digestive pole. To put it another way, the etheric forces which are at the service of the physical body in the metabolic-limb system have been 'moved upwards' in the nerve-sense system and put to the service of the astral body and, to some extent, of the Ego. This does not mean that the upper and lower poles work in opposition to one another in the healthy human being. Rather, they work together, mediated by the rhythmic system, in complementary harmony with one another. How this supposedly happens can be illustrated by Rudolf Steiner's explanation of the processes which follow the individual's consumption of food of either plant or animal origin.

Mankind cannot, of course, live without eating. Yet all food is, in some ways, alien to the human organism, for it is saturated with its native etheric forces, qualitatively different from those of the system into which they have been ingested. During digestion, said Steiner, two quite different series of processes are being carried on. The first series is the physical digestion of food in the normal ways such as are described in textbooks of human physiology: starches are broken down into glucose, proteins into their constituent aminoacids and so on. The second series is of an astral-etheric nature, the ingested food being stripped of its extra-human etheric forces by means of the influence of astral forces emanating from the cephalic pole. After the simpler substances into which ingested food has been broken down have been absorbed into the body through the walls of the stomach and the intestines, they are humanized by other astral forces emanating from the motor-digestive pole, which imbue them with native etheric force. Thus what are, in the context of digestion, the breaking-down functions of the cephalic pole and the building-up functions of the metabolic pole work in harmony towards the same end, the absorption of alien substances into the human biosystem.

It will be remembered that at the cephalic pole etheric forces (similar to those which, at the metabolic pole, are concerned with cellular regeneration and replacement) are transmuted into thought and memory. What happens to them in the rhythmic system, the respiratory and circulatory processes which mediate, like a perpetually swinging pendulum, between the two poles? To some extent, said Steiner, they became bound up into the emotional life of the individual, which can be looked upon as a psychic breathing. For just as breathing can be broken down into a rhythmic alternation between inspiration and expiration, so the emotional life alternates between sympathy and antipathy, attraction and repulsion.

The consciousness of the healthy human being is normally unaware, or very little aware, of the complex processes which are going on within it. We do not feel, in the nerve-sense application of the word, digestion taking place or the kidneys carrying out their functions. Conscious awareness of these processes only arises when something is going wrong: when we feel the processes of digestion is when they are not proceeding normally, the times when we complain of flatulence, heartburn or indigestion.

Anthroposophical physicians attach much significance to this. They say that consciousness, in which both the ego and the astral body are particularly involved, properly pertains to the cephalic pole and the nerve-sense system; when it is transferred to, or developed within, the metabolic pole and motor-digestive system, or when it manifests itself in the activities of the rhythm system, it is a clear indication of illness or, at best, some disorder which could eventually result in illness.

Such disorders may have many *immediate* causes, of which the successful invasion of the body by outside life forms —

bacteria, fungi or parasites, for example – is the most obvious instance. But what is it that causes such an invasion to be successful in one human body and not in another? Steiner replied that only an organism in disequilibrium, an organism in which the etheric, astral and spiritual vehicles are not operating through and on the triune system as they should, is capable of being successfully invaded in this way. Whatever, he said, are the immediate causes, the ultimate causes of disease arise from imbalances between the forces of the Ego, the astral and etheric bodies, and the activities of the nerve-sense, rhythmic and metabolic systems.

As an example of a simple disorder producing no more than minor inconvenience arising from disequilibrium, students of anthroposophical medicine often instance the sort of cramps which many people experience at night, usually as they are drifting toward sleep. According to anthroposophical teaching, sleep is far more than a physiological process involving only a reduction of the level of brain activity. In human sleep the Ego and higher aspects of the astral body are believed to separate from the etheric and physical bodies; in other words, in sleep the sleeper approaches the state of an animal or even a plant. This does not mean, of course, that the activities of the cephalic pole completely cease – if they did, sleep would pass into coma and, eventually, death – but it does mean that its activity is greatly reduced, and that it is temporarily outside the control of the Ego and the higher astral forces which are associated with it.

As the Ego begins and carries through its withdrawal from association with the etheric/physical complex, the nerve-sense processes which are centred at the cephalic pole are still very active but are no longer properly directed. In these circumstances it is sometimes the case that they encroach upon the metabolic-limb system, particularly on any part of it which has been weakened or made more sensitive to outside influences by age or injury, inducing the phenomena associated with night cramps. The pain from these jerks the sleeper into awakeness or, in anthroposophical terminology, reunites the Ego and its associated astral forces with the physical and etheric bodies. This reunion often leads to a fairly quick cessation of the cephalic pole's intrusion into the metabolic-limb system and a consequent diminution in the intensity of the cramp – which, alas, often recurs as sleep approaches and the Ego renews its withdrawal.

A far more painful condition supposedly resulting from forces which should be active at one pole being at work in the other is migraine, which is largely the outcome, so it is said, of a morbid diminution at the cephalic pole of activities relating to the Ego and the astral body. This belief does not imply that the *immediate* causes of the symptoms of migraine are not physiological changes in the physical body. What is asserted is that such changes result from the incorrect functioning of the Ego and the astral body.

Anything, so anthroposophical physicians maintain, which causes an excessive reduction in astral and spiritual (i.e. related to the Ego) activity at the cephalic pole can result in an attack of migraine. One of the most frequent causes of such a reduction, however, relates to the non-material aspects of the processes which take place in the gastro-intestinal tract. It will be remembered that Steiner claimed that these exhibited a dual action of astral forces – those emanating from the cephalic pole stripping the ingested food of extra-human etheric forces, those from the metabolic pole imbuing the broken-down food with etheric forces native to humanity. If, however, some factor such as stress, overwork or the reception of an excessive flow of sense impressions (all of which, whatever their source, are processed by the nerve-sense system which is concentrated at the cephalic pole) makes very large demands on the cephalic pole, there results in inadequate transference of astral energies to the digestive system and, as a consequence of this, substances enter the blood stream which have not been completely stripped of formative forces which are of plant or animal origin. The organism, desperate to restore normality, endeavours to deal with the situation by further depleting the cephalic pole of its astral and spiritual energies – already insufficient to deal with stress or other triggering factors – and to 'digest' the alien substances in the organs of the nerve-sense system, which were not intended for that purpose. Such an unnatural endeavour causes too close an association between the Ego, which initiates it, and the organs in question, and acute pain – the classic migraine – results.

Migraine seems to occur more frequently in women than in men, a divergence which is partly explicable by Rudolf Steiner's claim that the Ego and the astral body act more intensely at the motor-digestive pole in the female sex than in the male, the position being reversed where the cephalic pole is concerned. Some anthroposophical physicians have argued that other factors in this sexual divergence are related to menstrual disorders.

The late Dr Ita Wegman, a pioneer in the development of the medical aspects of anthroposophy, gave details of an interesting case history which seems of much relevance in this context. Dr Wegman's patient, who came to the anthroposophical clinic at Arlesheim in Switzerland at the age of fifty-five, had suffered for twenty years from regular attacks of migraine, the frequency being about one attack every three to four weeks. At the age of forty she had undergone a hysterectomy, following which the migraine attacks increased in both intensity and duration, and from her forty-sixth year onwards produced such prolonged periods of pain that she sometimes lost consciousness. Other symptoms of the patient's general malaise were a frequency of micturition amounting almost to chronic cystitis, insomnia and a constant lassitude of such severity that the patient 'woke up feeling tired'.

Most Swiss physicians of the time would have been inclined (as they still are) to consider the constant tiredness as a classic symptom of clinical depression and to regard the migraine and other symptoms of ill health as being of exclusively psychological origin. The diagnosis arrived at by Dr Wegman in collaboration with Rudolf Steiner – and almost certainly owing to the latter's employment of supposed higher modes of perception – was very different. The action of the Ego, it was decided, was weak and unable properly to control the etheric and astral forces relating to the metabolic pole. As a consequence of this, the effects of processes which properly pertained to the metabolic-limb system had penetrated the nerve-sense system. The etheric and astral forces of the metabolic pole were operating largely independently of the Ego and, as a consequence, were inducing excessive activity in some parts of the organism. For example, the kidneys, which, as will be subsequently explained, are believed to have a particular and close relationship with the astral body, performed their functions with such enthusiasm that the frequency of micturition became pathological. As for the insomnia and the consequent fatigue, this, said Dr Wegman, was caused by the weak Ego having difficulty in drawing the astral forces away from their close bonding to the physical and etheric bodies. Anthroposophists, it will be remembered, believe that such a temporary separation always accompanies healthy sleep. The increasing intensity of migraine headaches following hysterectomy was attributed to astral forces associated with the reproductive system acting elsewhere in the organism without the proper control by the Ego.

The treatment given to the patient in question illustrates the holistic, dialectical approach associated with anthroposophical medicine – holistic, because it endeavours to treat the patient, the whole man or woman, rather than the disease; dialectical, because it is held that not only is the physical body influenced by non-material etheric, astral and spiritual forces, but that processes locked and frozen into physical substances can influence the Ego and other higher aspects of the human totality. On the basis of the diagnosis it was decided that it was essential that the Ego's capacity for penetrating its influence into the etheric and physical bodies should be strengthened. To this end, and presumably on the basis of indications given by Steiner, the treatment given included the application of herbal infusions derived from lime blossom and stinging nettles to the stomach and feet respectively. The nettle infusion, applied in the morning, was given with the object of facilitating the Ego's task of making the physical/etheric penetration which should follow sleep, while the lime-blossom infusion was intended to keep such penetration fully operative throughout the day. It was decided that, as the migraine attacks were believed to have largely resulted from the effects of astral forces particularly associated with the reproductive system, it was appropriate to administer extract of the root *Potentilla tormentilla* (tormentil, the herb of which English folk names include septfoil, bloodroot and thormantle) in highly potentized (or dynamized) form. Potentization techniques are fully described in the succeeding chapter. They are intended to unlock processes which are believed to be 'frozen' both into natural forms of minerals and into substances derived from animals and plants. According to Dr Wegman, her patient responded favourably to this surprising and highly unorthodox therapy.

At the present day remedies most commonly prescribed for migraine by anthroposophical physicians include Bidor, Ferr. Sulf. comp. and feverfew, a variety of chrysanthemum. Bidor is compounded from a formula devised by Steiner himself. It consists of iron sulphate, silica and honey, usually in the proportions 54:17:29; the second is, when reduced to its constituent chemical elements, very similar in composition to the first and contains dynamized sulphur, iron and quartz (natural silica); the last is also normally administered in dynamized form and seems to be a comparatively recent addition to the *materia medica* which makes up the therapeutic armoury of the anthroposophical practitioner.

The rationale for the employment of Bidor is as follows: the iron in iron sulphate stimulates the respiratory and circulation systems, and the sulphur activates the entire metabolism. Silica intensifies the processes which are concerned with form. The honey produces a response from the forces of the Ego. Save for the absence of honey, the make-up of Ferr. Sulf. comp. is essentially the same and the rationale underlying its therapeutic use is similar. In its dynamized form feverfew, which is not normally administered in the practice of anthroposophical medicine in the comparatively large doses which have been employed by traditional herbalists and orthodox physicians, is held by some to enable the Ego to control more easily processes pertaining to both the cephalic and metabolic poles.

In the course of reading my summary of Dr Wegman's treatment of her migraine patient it will probably have surprised some to note that she assumed that there was a specific association between the kidneys and the astral body — for, as stated on p. 38, the astral body pertains to the element of Air, while, from their specific excretory function, the kidneys might perhaps be expected to relate to elemental Water. In fact, all the elemental rulerships of the 'cardinal organs' of the human body — heart, lungs, liver and kidneys — are somewhat unexpected but, in the context of Rudolf Steiner's medical teachings, quite reasonable.

Steiner gave these elemental attributions in a lecture delivered at Dornach, Switzerland, on 2 July 1921. He said:

The lungs, as inner organ or organic system, contain the compressed coercive thoughts with all that we receive and concentrate in that organ through perception of outer objects. The liver has an entirely different relationship to the outer world. Because the lungs preserve the thought material they are quite differently shaped [from the liver]. They [the lungs] are more closely connected with the element of Earth. The liver, which conceals in particular the quietly appearing hallucinations, is connected with the element of Water, and the kidney system, paradoxical as it sounds, belongs to the element of Air. Naturally one thinks that this ought to be the case with the lungs, but *as organs* the lungs are connected with the element of Earth, although not with it alone. On the other hand the kidneys, *as organs*, belong to the element of Air, and the heart to warmth [Fire], being entirely composed out of that element. Hence this element [of Fire], which is the spiritual one, is the one which takes up the predisposition of our karma into the delicate warmth structure of the warmth organism.

Since the human being as a whole stands in a relationship with the exterior world you can readily realize that the lungs have a particular relationship to that exterior world in connection to the element of Earth and the liver in regard to the element of Water. If you examine the Earth qualities of plants you will find in them the remedies for diseases which originate in the lungs. . . . If you take what circulates in the plant, its juices, you will have the remedy for all disturbances connected with the liver. Thus a study of the reciprocal relationships between the organs and the exterior world offers, in fact, the foundations of a rational therapy.[2]

The teachings given in the above passage are correlated with anthroposophical beliefs concerning the correct elemental associations of the various components of the human organism in the following table.

Element	Human component	Cardinal organs
Fire	Ego (spirit)	Heart
Air	Astral ('emotional') body	Kidneys
Water	Etheric (formative) body	Liver
Earth	Physical body	Lungs

The first of these cardinal organs is described in the above quotation as being 'entirely composed' of warmth, that is, in the language of the ancients, elemental Fire. By this statement Rudolf Steiner was not, of course, intending to convey the absurd idea that he believed the heart to be made of physical material in the process of violent combustion. Rather was he intending to communicate to his listeners his belief that the *functions* of the heart, including those subtle functions he had perceived as a result of his use of the faculty of Intuition, are in essence derived from the world of the spirit in which the Ego has its existence. The heart, it could be said, shadows forth a physical image of the world of spirit forces and, in a similar fashion, the liver shadows forth the etheric world and the kidneys the astral world.

On a more immediate level – one that is of more particular relevance to anthroposophical medicine and the techniques its practitioners apply – the heart is seen as the organ at which the polarities of the nerve-sense and metabolic-limb systems have their meeting and, through the rhythmic system, equilibrate their forces. For anthroposophists the heart is to the body as the sun is to the solar system, the central source of warmth and light, the giver of equilibrium to the system as a whole. As such it is regarded as being, save where there is some congenital defect of the type which anthroposophists consider to be the final result of unbalanced etheric forces, *in its own essential nature* perfect; consequently, the causes of heart disease are always to be sought outside the heart itself.

Anthroposophical physicians, following Steiner's indications, have classified these external factors into a number of categories. To some extent these overlap with one another and, in the final analysis, they meld into one, a morbid predominance of the forces of either the cephalic or the metabolic pole. This is held to be the case even when the immediate cause of heart disease is probably some infectious disease, such as diphtheria or scarlet fever.

There is some disagreement amongst physiologists as to whether the concepts of a 'normal rate of heartbeat' or a 'normal rate of respiration' are meaningful. Most anthroposophical physicians, however, argue that, whatever wide variations there may be between one individual and another, there is a sort of 'Platonic ideal' of these rates and that these are invariably the rates exhibited by a human being whose entire organism is functioning as it should on every level of being. These ideal rates are 72 beats a minute for the heart, the indicator of the regular pulsations of the entire rhythmic system, and a quarter of that figure, 18 a minute, for the rate of respiration. There is a certain amount of empirical evidence that these are indeed the approximate rates which are to be observed in most healthy human beings who are neither over exerting themselves nor in a state of partial or complete somnolence. However, it seems that Rudolf Steiner, who attached a very considerable importance to these rates as indicators of the harmony between man and the cosmos, was impressed not so much by the empirical evidence derived from observation as by the fact that these rates have a certain consonance with both the life span of humanity and the solar cycle of time which the ancients named the 'Great Year'.

Steiner seems to have begun by calculating the 'ideal' number of heartbeats in a twenty-four-hour period as follows:

$$
\begin{array}{rl}
72 & \text{(number of heartbeats in a minute)} \\
\times\ 60 & \text{(minutes in one hour)} \\
\hline
4320 & \text{(number of heartbeats on one hour)} \\
\times\ 24 & \text{(hours in one day and night)} \\
\hline
103680 & \text{(heartbeats in one twenty-four-hour period)}
\end{array}
$$

He then divided this number by 4 — 4 being of numerical significance in relation to the human organism because of the four cardinal organs, the four temperaments, the four elements, etc. — which gives 25920, the number of 'ideal' cycles of respiration ($18 \times 60 \times 24$) in a day and a night.

Then, taking the 'ideal' lifespan of the human being as seventy-two solar years (seventy-two was an important number in kabbalistic numerology and there are continual references in Jewish mystical literature to the seventy-two names of God), he calculated the number of occasions on which a human being would undergo a sleep/wake cycle during a lifetime (365×72) on the assumption that there was only one period of full sleep, with withdrawal of the Ego and upper astral forces from the physical/etheric complex, in each twenty-four-hour period. The result (26280) is within 1.4 per cent of the respiration total of 25,980. Steiner saw this as more than coincidence and said:

You make in the course of your life as many inspirations and exhalations of the astral body and the Ego as you make daily in your respiratory inhalations and exhalations. These rhythms correspond absolutely, and show us how man is fitted into the cosmos. The life of one day . . . as a single circuit corresponds with the inner day that endures from birth to death.[3]

It seems that Steiner, like a number of other esotericists of his own time and since, attached a major significance to the fact that the approximate number of both daily respirations and lifetime sleep/wake cycles – around 26,000 – is more or less the same as the number of solar years, from one spring equinox to the next, in the Great Year. A Great Year is the period of time in which the moving, tropical zodiac performs one complete revolution of 360 degrees in relation to the fixed, sidereal zodiac which is based on the constellations.[4]

Such numerological considerations – I do not use the phrase in any pejorative sense – undoubtedly reinforced Steiner's belief, based on both tradition and his own clairvoyant perceptions, that the idea of a relationship between the sun and the human heart was far more than a poetic fancy. As is described in the succeeding chapter, a belief in this and similar relationships between particular bodily organs and constituent parts of our solar system has had pharmacological and therapeutic implications for the development of anthroposophical medicine.

As was said earlier, anthroposophical physicians look

upon the ultimate source of all afflictions of the body's central sun, the heart, as being a disequilibrium between the cephalic and metabolic poles and associated forces. Endocarditis and pericarditis are said to be typical of disorders arising from a disequilibrium caused by metabolic predominance. Cardiac infarction and angina pectoris are regarded as being equally typical of exactly the opposite malfunction, a cephalic predominance. In the former case the infections which are directly responsible for the disease are believed to be encouraged by proteins which, owing to cephalic deficiency, have been insufficiently 'humanized' before being incorporated into the structure of the heart; in the latter case the immediate cause, which leads up to a heart attack – the narrowing of the arteries – is said to be a consequence of an excess of the hardening, sclerosing forces which are associated with the actions of the nerve-sense system centred on the cephalic pole.

Rudolf Steiner, like C. G. Jung, considered the ancient concept of the four temperaments, in accordance with which individuals are psychophysically classified into groups associated with the four elements, to be still applicable in the twentieth century. For reasons difficult to fathom, however, he made some minor but confusing changes in the traditional terminology, so his use of such words as 'sanguine' (or 'choleric') may not be quite the same as the words when used by other writers. Steiner's choleric man is the man in whom the heart (and that which particularly relates to it, the Ego) is dominant. The Emperor Napoleon, said Steiner, was an almost archetypal representative of the choleric (Fire) temperament – psychologically strong, inflexibly pursuing his aims, generous when generosity suited his purposes and prone to anger. To this it might be added that when this temperament expresses itself pathologically one gets an Adolf Hitler rather than a Napoleon Bonaparte.

Steiner's sanguine, or nervous, human being contrasts very markedly with his choleric category. While in the choleric, or heart, individual it is the Ego and the forces of Fire which are predominant, in the nervous individual it is the astral body and Air, both associated with the kidneys. The astral body expresses itself in the emotional life, and the emotional life of the (nervous or sanguine) individual is subject — like the winds, expressions of the Air principle — to sudden changes of direction, to violent turbulence succeeded by calm. Sanguine men or women are thus subject to indecision and mood changes of such violence that, at times, they appear almost schizoid. Such variability extends itself from the emotional life to the physical. At one time such people may exhibit frenzied activity which is rapidly followed, perhaps only moments later, by laziness verging on apathy. There is an Air-like intellectual tendency which flares up and down but does not burn with the power and consistency of the 'hard gem-like flame' of the choleric man or woman.

One of the terms ascribed by Steiner to the temperament of the kidney person is 'sanguine', an adjective derived from the Latin word for 'blood'. The kidneys, in fact, have a particular relationship with arterial blood, bright red and oxygen-charged, and, according to Steiner, oxygen is the physical medium through which the astral body acts in collaboration with etheric forces to initiate anabolic, building-up, processes. He said that the raw materials of anabolic processes, the substances derived from food and stripped of extra-human etheric forces in the digestive tract, are assimilated into the human biosystem — impregnated with native, human astrality — by a 'radiation' centred on the kidneys which extends throughout the entire organism. For anthroposophical physicians, then, the kidneys have a dual function. Not only are they organs of excretion, a process which Steiner believed had its origins in astral activity taking place through the nerve-sense system, but they are organs of assimilation.

Steiner's views on the functions of the liver, which he believed to be the organ peculiarly and particularly associated with elemental Water and the etheric body, were equally unorthodox. The liver, he said, not only carried out all the biochemical processes known to physiologists, for example the manufacture of fat from surplus glucose, but was the centre of etheric activity which ultimately controlled all the 'water processes' of the body; furthermore, there was, so he claimed, a plantlike quality to some of the liver's activities, which he compared to those of leaves.

He also, in accordance with traditional beliefs, associated the liver with the phlegmatic temperament, the man or woman in whom the ever-flowing forces of the etheric body are dominant. These flowing streams of etheric Water tend to find their own level, and the psychologically healthy phlegmatic individual is like a calm inland lake: ripples, even waves, sometimes disturb its surface, but soon all returns to normal and all is once again placid. This placidity can, in certain cases, become pathological, and the phlegmatic man becomes a depressive – not, however, always a manic depressive, for the depression suffered by Steiner's liver man or woman can be a continuous and, in a sense, sodden apathy.

The structure and functions of the lungs would suggest to most people that they pertained to the Air element, but Rudolf Steiner, who saw them as the cardinal organs which most closely express the whole nature of the physical body and its relationship with dense matter, ascribed them to Earth. While this rather surprising teaching is undoubtedly based on Steiner's own use of the unusual modes of perception which were available to him – and, perhaps, indications given by such writers on occult medicine as Papus – he provided for it something approaching an empirical rationale. The lungs, he said, show their close relationship to the physical world by the fact that, through the processes of respiration, they are not only in continual contact with the world of matter, in the forms of oxygen, nitrogen and other gases, but are always in process of taking parts of that matter into themselves and making it available to the physical body. This applies, Steiner correctly pointed out, even when exhalation is in progress. Furthermore, by their continual involvement in the body's oxygen/haemoglobin/carbon dioxide cycle they indicate a special relationship with the mineral carbonates which can be taken as typical manifestations of the Earth element.

The temperament associated with the lungs by Steiner is that of the melancholic – in this context the word does not always imply depression – the man or woman whose personal characteristics suggest the qualities of elemental Earth, such as weight, solidity and apartness from the rest of creation. In its pathological form, said Steiner, this temperament can manifest itself in conditions in which agoraphobia and other anxiety states are combined with depression.

The outline I have given of Rudolf Steiner's teachings concerning, first, the nature of the mineral, plant and animal kingdoms and, secondly, 'the kingdom of man', the human organism with its four cardinal organs, its poles equilibrated by the rhythmic system, and its physical, etheric and astral bodies, illustrates the extraordinarily complex theoretical structure which underlies the practice of anthroposophical medicine and pharmacy.

Regardless of the truth or falsehood of the structure as a whole, there are two important points which I believe should be held in mind. The first concerns something that to some seems to be *missing* from the structure, in spite of its complexity; the second concerns the provenance, as it were, of the theoretical underpinnings of anthroposophical medicine and, indeed, the anthroposophical world picture as a whole.

What is missing from Steiner's account of the human totality and from any anthroposophical texts published subsequent to his death in 1925 – or what, at any rate, seems to be missing to many of those who have studied anthroposophical literature – is any attempt to incorporate even heavily modified forms of the concepts associated with the various schools of modern depth psychology into the theoretical structure of anthroposophy. This is particularly surprising as at least some of those concepts, even those which at first sight appear excessively materialistic, appear to the outside observer to be in general conformity with Steiner's teachings and, furthermore, actually strengthen the case for anthroposophy.

It seems virtually certain that this situation has arisen as a result of the fact that such concepts are bound up with theories concerning the existence and functioning of the Unconscious. As was described in the preceding chapter, as a young man Rudolf Steiner had rejected with utter revulsion the pessimistic philosophy of von Hartmann, a philosophy which was based on a particular theory concerning unconscious, instinctive drives. So great was Steiner's reaction against this philosophy that until the very end of his life he virtually refused to accept the existence of any meaningful psychology in which the concept of the Unconscious played an important part. A lecture he gave in 1917 illustrates this attitude. He said:

Jung was led to posit two unconscious minds, the first being the individual unconscious, concealed within [and peculiar to] the individual human being. If in her childhood the young woman [referred to earlier] jumped out of a carriage and received a shock the incident has long since vanished from consciousness, but survives subconsciously. If you consider this subconscious element, made up of innumerable details, you get the personal, or individual, Unconscious. This is the first of Jung's differentiations.

But the second is the *Collective* Unconscious. He says: 'There are things affecting the life of the psyche which exist neither in the [individual] personality nor in the objectively existing exterior world, and which must therefore be accepted as psychic realities.'

The aim of psychoanalysis is to bring such psychic content into consciousness. That is supposedly the healing technique, to bring everything into consciousness. Thus the physician must undertake to bring forth from the patient, not only what he has experienced from birth onwards, but what has no objective existence and therefore has to be presumed as existing in the psychic world. . . . This has driven the psychoanalyst to say that a man thus experiences not only what happens to him after his physical birth, but also all sorts of things which preceded his birth. . . . A man who is born today . . . experiences the Greek gods, the whole past of mankind. The evil of this is the fact that he experiences it subconsciously. . . . It growls like demons.

. . . if [the psychoanalyst] is true to his theory [he] would have to take these things seriously and simply say that when a man grows up and may be made ill by his relationship to that which stirs within him . . . it must be explained to him that there is a spiritual world inhabited by various gods.

. . . Jung . . . goes so far as to assert that the gods . . . become angry and revenge themselves, this revenge showing itself as hysteria. Very well, it amounts then to this; such a contemporary man who is mistreated by a demon in his unconscious mind, does not know there are demons and cannot achieve any conscious relationship with them because to do so would be superstitious.

. . . so you see the present-day physician is forced to say to himself: 'Men are tormented by spirits, and because they are taught nothing about them ... they ... project their demons out- wards. . . .' Jung . . . says: 'Certain of my colleagues claim that the psychic energies that spring from such torment must be delivered into another course . . . [but] it is not always possible to divert this energy. . . .' . . . the psychoanalyst . . . says to himself . . . 'For God's sake . . . do not let us take the spiritual world seriously.' It does not enter their minds to take the spiritual world seriously. Then something very peculiar happens. . . . I shall read to you [from Jung's *Psychology of the Unconscious*]: 'The primeval pictures [which make up the contents of the Collective Uncon- scious] contain not only the best and greatest of all that mankind has felt, but also every infamous and devilish deed of which men have been capable. The mistake [the patient] makes . . . is attribu- ting to himself the contents of the Collective Unconscious. . . . Here lies the psychological reason why men have always needed demons and were never able to live without gods. . . .'

Thus, you see . . . the psychoanalyst ridicules men. . . . The psychoanalyst proves to you that man becomes ill and useless without his God, but says that this need has nothing to do with the existence or non-existence of God.

Considered as a whole, the lecture from which I have quoted the above is a diatribe aimed at Jung's *Psychology of the Unconscious*, a book to which the overworked adjective 'seminal' can, I think, be properly applied. In a later chapter I shall endeavour to show that Rudolf Steiner's rejection of Jungian depth psychology was based on a failure to fully understand that psychology, a confusion between Jung's Collective Unconscious and the 'instinctive unconscious' of von Hartmann. At this stage it is sufficient to note as a fact that, rightly or wrongly, Steiner rejected any psychological concept which he considered as in some way reducing the individual's responsibility for his or her own actions, his or her spiritual freedom.

The second point which I believe should be held in mind in considering the theoretical structure which underlies anthroposophical therapies concerns their origins, their provenance.

It is a curious fact that an identical mistake about the nature of these origins has been made by three groups of people: those who regard Rudolf Steiner as having been a schizophrenic; those who regard him as having been a charlatan; and those enthusiasts who have such an uncritical admiration for Steiner's work that they are unable to admit that he was in any way influenced by his contemporaries or, indeed, any writer much later than Goethe. It is only fair to say that, on the basis of personal observation, I believe this latter group to include only a very small proportion of those who would regard themselves as committed anthroposophists. The mistake in question is to believe that Rudolf Steiner's teachings, or even the greater part of those teachings, originated with him and should be regarded, as the first group would insist, as a remarkably coherent and internally consistent delusional system, or should be looked upon as an elaborate series of lies designed to bolster up a mystical confidence trick, or, as the group of uncritical devotees seem to believe, must be assumed to be almost totally derived from Steiner's employment of supernormal faculties of perception.

The fact is, however, that while the *form* in which Steiner expressed his teachings was largely his own, a very large proportion of the *content* of those teachings – perhaps as much as 75–80 per cent – was familiar to, and commonly accepted by, the generality of Western occultists long before Steiner began, in 1900, to lecture in public on such matters. This applies to not only such widespread concepts as those of the existence of the astral and other subtle bodies, the idea of the psychophysical temperaments and their correspondence with the elements of Earth, Air, Fire and Water, the existence of the spagyric principles of salt, sulphur and mercury, and so on. It is equally applicable to Steiner's exposition of the triune division of the human organism into two poles and an equilibriating rhythm system which, as pointed out earlier, is more or less identical, in spite of terminological differences, with the classification advocated by Papus, the French occult physician. As was stated in the preceding chapter, it was by extending this system to a consideration of society as a whole that were evolved both the synarchy of Saint-Yves and the concept of the threefold commonwealth which was of such concern to Rudolf Steiner in, particularly, the years 1916–22. Even the idea of 'kidney radiation', that the kidneys have an assimilative function connected with astralization processes, often asserted to be originated by Steiner – and cerainly unfamiliar to the medical audience to which he expounded it – is to be found in some pre-1900 books on the subject of occult medicine.

This does *not* mean that Steiner was entirely unoriginal, a mere systematizer of familiar occult concepts; nor does it mean that he did not possess the faculties of perception by Imagination, Inspiration and Intuition. It does mean, however, that he was a link – perhaps a uniquely important link – in a chain of esoteric tradition which extends backwards into history and forwards into the future, not some one true Prophet.

I am inclined to believe that Rudolf Steiner had access, as he claimed to have had access, to higher modes of perception – although I suspect that his perceptions were more subject to error than the majority of anthroposophists would be prepared to accept – and that with the use of these he came to his conclusions as to how far traditional esoteric beliefs were either acceptable as they stood or were in need of modification and/or amplification. This is not to say that some aspects of anthroposophical thought in general and anthroposophical medicine in particular, did not very largely come into existence in a systematized form as the result of Steiner's use of his perceptive faculties; a case in point is anthroposophical pharmacy, which I describe in my next chapter.

3

Towards a New Pharmacology

A common dictionary definition of a polymath is 'one who understands many arts and sciences'. No one who has more than the slightest acquaintance with the writings of Rudolf Steiner can doubt that he was such a person. But Steiner was far more than a polymath: he was a major interdisciplinary scholar, a man whose learning and insight enabled him to cross the barriers that compartmentalize the sciences and the arts into seeming isolation from one another. The extraordinarily varied audiences to whom he addressed his lectures – farmers, physicians and trade unionists, for example – were enabled to see that their especial interests were part of a much greater whole, a living unity which subsumed them all.

Steiner was a man who spoke and wrote with authority, but he did not approach his students as some sort of authoritarian guru, a spiritual and intellectual dictator laying down, in infinite detail, precise instructions as to how they should conduct their personal lives, their farms and gardens, their medical practices and so on. Instead he acted as have all the most stimulating and creative teachers, making every effort to do no more than provide guidelines and pointers which could be applied and developed by the pupils themselves. Only by such self-development, considered Steiner, could both the individual human being and society as a whole gain any real and lasting benefits from the application of the insights provided by spiritual science to the business of everyday life.

This approach was typified by Steiner's teachings on the subject of the medicaments to be used by the anthroposophical physician in his or her endeavours to extend the healing art. He did not proclaim some new, fully developed 'spiritual pharmacology' by which medicaments were ordered to be manufactured and administered in accordance with mechanically rigid rules by robot-like pharmacists and physicians. What he did was to give, usually in the context of actual cases, broad indications of possible remedies and their preparation. It was the task of his medical pupils to take such indications as no more than hypotheses, subject to amendment or abandonment as impractical, incomplete or even erroneous, and to work out their therapeutic and pharmacological implications for themselves.

The preparation of a particular medicament is considered to be of enormous importance by practitioners of anthroposophical medicine. It is held that there is a real difference, not detectable by even the most refined methods of chemical analysis but significant in terms of therapeutic efficacy, between a remedy, such as a plant extract, which has been prepared in accordance with the techniques developed by anthroposophical physicians and pharmacists and one which has not. These techniques are similar to, but by no means identical with, some of the techniques used in the preparation of homoeopathic medicines; thus, for example, many anthroposophical remedies are administered, like homoeopathic medicines, in 'dynamized' or 'potentized' form.

In essence dynamization, as practised by such manufacturers of anthroposophic pharmaceutical products as the Swiss manufacturer WALA and the worldwide Weleda group of associated companies, is simple enough. A medicinal raw material, perhaps a solution of some metallic salt or a plant extract, is added to some inert substance in the proportion of 1 in 10 and thoroughly mixed with it, most usually by succussion, that is, shaking and banging. It is normal to give at least a hundred succussions. For these the mixture is placed in a firmly corked or stoppered container and each time the container is shaken its base is banged against some firm but elastic surface (the first writer to describe the process in print used a leatherbound book for the purpose). At the end of the first succussion process the resulting product consists, of course, of a 1 in 10 mixture of the original substance and its dilutant, usually water or grain spirit.[1] This is referred to as the 'first decimal potency', commonly abbreviated to either 1x or, in continental Europe, 1D.

The process is then repeated with one part of the 1x material to nine parts of dilutant, producing the second decimal potency (2x), one part of the 2x material to nine parts of dilutant, producing the third decimal potency (3x), and so on, until the desired degree of potentization has been achieved.[2] Sometimes the process is continued until the thirtieth decimal potency (30x), but long before that stage has been reached *the original substance has ceased to be contained in the potentized medicament*; it can be mathematically demonstrated that on a molecular level no part of the raw material can be present at potencies above 23x.

This has led critics of potentization to assert that those who prescribe medicines prepared in this way are administering totally inert substances to their patients. Any beneficial effects resulting from their use can only, so it is said, be the result of the 'placebo effect' – the patient getting better because he believes that the medicine he has taken will make him better.

Anthroposophical physicians and others who employ potentized remedies do not agree. They argue that any natural substance of the sort used as the raw material of potentized remedies is more than a mere collection of molecules of greater or lesser complexity. Be it a naturally occurring ore, such as cinnabar or pyrites, a mineral substance of organic origin, such as ground oyster shell, or a plant extract, it carries latent within it the essence of the cosmic and telluric (earthly) processes that brought it into being. Successive succussions or, in the case of insoluble solids, grindings supposedly release the 'essential natures' of these processes *and imprint them upon the inert dilutants*. By definition the content of such 'process imprintings' could not be amenable to chemical analysis. Just as chemical analysis of the paper on which a Shakespeare sonnet was written can give no indication of the emotional, intellectual or spiritual content of that sonnet, so a chemical analysis of a highly potentized remedy can give no indication of its process content and its therapeutic effects. In short, such medicaments are possessed of immaterial qualities.

The belief that highly dynamized or potentized medicaments are possessed of qualities pertaining to non-material modes of being did not originate with anthroposophic medicine. In his *Organon of Healing*, the first edition of which was published some fifty years before the birth of Rudolf Steiner, Samuel Hahnemann, the founder of modern homoeopathy, referred to what he called 'the spiritlike' characteristics of potentized medicines. He claimed such dynamizations develop

the inner, spirit-like medicinal powers of crude substances to an unheard of degree and make all of them exceedingly, immeasurably, penetrating, active and effective – even those that in the raw state do not have the slightest medicinal effect . . . there is a natural law by which . . . forces capable of altering the health of living organisms are generated in the raw material of a remedy through the use of trituration [rubbing or grinding to a fine powder], and succussion. . . .

This remarkable transformation of the properties of natural substances . . . develops latent dynamic powers previously imperceptible and, as it were, lying hidden and asleep . . . by the trituration of a medicinal substance and the succussion of its solution . . . the material is spiritualized, if one may use the expression. . . .

. . . trituration and succussion unlock the natural substances, uncover and reveal the specific medicinal powers lying hidden in their souls. The dilutant is only an auxiliary, although indispensable, factor.

. . . the medicinal substance that seems to us only crude matter . . . is . . . completely transformed and refined by . . . progressive dynamizations to become a spirit-like medicinal force.

. . . It is highly probable that during such dynamization . . . the material substance eventually dissolves completely into its individual spirit-like essence. . . .

This spirit-like medicinal power . . . is no longer perceptible to the senses . . . but demonstrates its power in the sick organism.

Anthroposophical physicians insist, as did Hahnemann, that highly dynamized medicines with a potency above 23x are, indeed, effective and that their patients have benefited from their use in a way that cannot be explained by the placebo effect. Such evidence is, of course, anecdotal, and there are serious and perhaps insurmountable difficulties associated with the possible carrying out of comparative clinical trials. Curiously enough, however, there is some botanical evidence for the efficacy of mineral salts administered in dynamizations so high – up to 60x – that no molecular traces of these minerals' original substance can be present.

This evidence was produced as the result of experimental work carried out by the late Dr Lili Kolisko, who put into practice a suggestion made by Rudolf Steiner that seeds should be germinated under exposure to dynamized minerals and the growth of the resulting plants should be compared with the growth of plants grown under precisely the same conditions but without such exposure. Over a period of a quarter of a century or so Dr Kolisko carried out such experiments, recording her results as 'potency growth curves'. These curves, of which Dr Kolisko produced several hundred, seemed to show a statistically significant relationship with the administration of minerals in high dynamizations.

In practice medicaments of such high potencies as those with which Dr Kolisko carried out her botanical experiments are rarely employed by anthroposophical practitioners and it is unusual for potencies of more than 30x to be administered to patients. There are some exceptions to this: belladonna 60x, for example, has been found useful in the treatment of a wide variety of psychic upheavals and disturbances. It is almost always given subcutaneously, that is, by injection immediately below the surface of the skin rather than into muscular tissue or the bloodstream.

Subcutaneous injection of this sort is a feature of anthroposophical medical techniques and, for the administration of dynamized substances, is regarded as being often preferable to taking the same medicine by mouth. There are a number of reasons for this preference, the most important of them being that it is believed that the very abnormality of injection – the fact that it is not the normal mode by which the organism receives foreign substances into itself – results in the substance administered being more rapidly productive of some effect upon the biosystem into which it has been introduced. It is held that such injections are particularly desirable when the physician wishes to influence the body through the rhythmic system (see p. 41). Oral administration of remedial substances is regarded as more appropriate when it is the metabolic-limb system which is the chosen path to the biosystem, while externally applied medicaments, be they oils, ointments, lotions or even remedial baths, pertain most especially to the nerve-sense system.

Which of the three bodily systems – nerve, metabolic or rhythmic – the physician wishes a remedy to work upon to some extent determines the exact degree of dynamization of that remedy. As a broad rule of thumb it is accepted that fairly low dynamizations, that is, potencies below, say, 7x, have a pronounced effect upon the metabolic system; medium dynamizations, from 8x to 15x, act upon the rhythmic system; while high dynamizations, notably those above 23x, are extremely potent in their effects upon the nerve-sense system. In other words, to influence the subtle nerve-sense system it is considered desirable to use remedies in which the medicinal raw product is no longer present and all that remains is the inert dilutant bearing the imprint of cosmic and terrestrial processes.

The introductions of such highly dynamized medicaments into the human body is not considered by anthroposophical physicians to be in any way unnatural. It is contended that when a human being or an animal ingests food or drink a dynamization process inevitably follows – the organism potentizes everything taken into it, thus releasing for its own use the dynamic-process imprint of cosmic and earthly energies. The preparation of a dynamized medicament, on this hypothesis, relieves the patient's biosystem of the task of potentization, thus enabling a more rapid and effective assimilation of the remedy.

Dynamized medicaments derived from animals are used by anthroposophical physicians as well as those derived from minerals and plants. A very large number of such preparations, some derived from whole creatures such as the honey bee and the garden spider, others from particular mammalian organs, such as the heart or the pancreas, are now available. Most commonly, organ preparations are used homologically, that is, to treat the corresponding organ in the patient's body, but they are also sometimes used in combination with the potentized plant or mineral substances for the treatment of more general conditions. Thus, for example, for chronic weeping eczema the anthroposophical physician might prescribe an organ preparation derived from the pancreatic gland in combination with potentized equisetum, the common horsetail, while in some cases of severe shock he might administer the same organ preparation in combination with a mineral remedy, potentized meteoric iron.

Anthroposophical physicians and pharmacists do not despise traditional herbal wisdom, and they are not ashamed to say that in seeking indications of the possible medical value of a particular plant they sometimes use a variant of the old 'doctrine of signatures'. Believers in this doctrine, particularly associated with the name of Paracelsus but not invented by him, asserted that the colour, form and general appearance of a plant, or of part of a plant, provided a 'signature' which indicated to which diseased human organ it might be of benefit. Thus, for example, any seed or leaf which was vaguely heart-shaped would have been considered as a possible remedy for a diseased heart. Similarly walnut kernels, their convolutions and their divisions into right and left hemispheres vaguely suggestive of the structure of the brain, might have been considered as suitable remedies for those suffering from head injuries. In this crude form anthroposophical physicians are not, of course, devotees of the doctrine of signatures. They accept, nevertheless, that with the aid of higher modes of perception the shapes, colours, habitats and life cycles of plants can provide important indications of their therapeutic employment.

A good example of this approach is supplied by a consideration of the grounds on which anthroposophical physicians, following indications given by Rudolf Steiner, came to the conclusion that some preparation of mistletoe *might* prove a useful adjunct to such orthodox treatments for cancer as surgery, chemotherapy and radiation. The mistletoe is a most unusual plant. It never roots in the ground under its own impulse and, indeed, is quite incapable of doing so. Instead it sinks its suckers into the sap-carrying system of oaks, apples, elms and other trees. And yet it is not, so it would seem, a parasite in the ordinary sense of the word. Its relationship with its host is symbiotic – it takes water and mineral salts supplied by the tree on which it grows and, in return, supplies the host tree with sugars which it has manufactured by photosynthesis.

The form of the mistletoe is also unusual. The normal structure of any plant, from a buttercup to a mighty cedar, is vertical – its roots are buried in the earth, its stem or trunk rises above them, and it is surmounted by leaf, blossom and, at the appropriate time, fruit or seed. In other words, it is both geotropic and phototropic; its roots grow downwards, responding to the pull of gravity and other terrestrial forces, while its foliage grows upwards, seeking light or other cosmic influences. But the structure of a mistletoe plant is spherical rather than vertical. It grows into the shape of a roughly formed ball, much of its foliage lying below the level of its sucker and seemingly indifferent as to its orientation to the light.

Its mode of reproduction is also notably different from that of most other plants. It flowers towards the end of one winter and, in summer, bears green berries which only ripen in the next winter, at the coldest time of the year.

In short, it is the supreme individualist of the plant world, its life style suggesting independence from the forces of earth and heaven alike, its unnatural rhythms running counter to those of the rest of the vegetable kingdom.

Anthroposophical physicians do not regard all this as no more than mere botanical eccentricity. The life of the mistletoe, they say, is closed off from the influences of both the earth and, as represented by the rhythm of the seasons, the cosmos. And, as a consequence of this, its life is in every way the antithesis of that of a malignant growth which, so it is said, is in all ways open to the influences of the external forces which induce cell proliferation.

To appreciate this argument fully it is essential to understand that the anthroposophical interpretation of biology is opposed to the reductionist view that a living organism is no more than an aggregation of cells. The reductionist argues that as the cell is the basic unit of life all that is necessary to understand the nature of a living being and its disorders is to understand the cell and its pathology. Anthroposophists and others who take the holistic view that any protoplasmic entity, be it plant, animal or human being, is more than the sum of its parts, insist, in opposition to the reductionist view, that while the cell must be studied on a cellular and subcellular level it can only be fully understood when it is also considered as part of a greater whole, a dynamic system subject to continuous change and always in process of interaction with the external world.

A helpful analogy, which has found favour amongst anthroposophists, was made by Professor D. W. Smithers. The activities that go on within a living organism, he said, can be compared with a game of billiards, the individual cells being the balls with which the game is played. The rules governing the game, life, cannot be deduced from a study of the properties of the individual billiard ball, the cell. The rules of the game of billiards originated elsewhere than on the table on which the game is played and a billiard ball miraculously endowed with consciousness would have to consider them as either having spontaneously come into existence or as the manifestation of some 'invisible controlling force'. Just as an invisible controlling force, the rules of billiards, determine that billiard balls should be spherical and not egg-shaped so, argues anthroposophical medicine, invisible forces determine the structure and form of the cell.

It will be remembered (see p. 43) that anthroposophists regard two such invisible forces as being at work in any living system: the force which leads to growth and expansion and the force which limits and organizes that growth. In health, it is asserted, the growth and organizing forces are operating in balanced harmony. In cancer, however, the organizing processes, which are closely related to the quality of individuality, personal uniqueness, are weak, and the growth process has gone out of control. What is needed is a strengthening of the individuality of the patient, of the formative forces that are concerned with control, order and independence. These, of course, are precisely the qualities that the mistletoe seems to exhibit in its independence from terrestrial and cosmic influences.

On the basis of these analogies a preparation derived from mistletoe has been developed and is now manufactured and sold under the name Iscador. It must be emphasized that Iscador is *not* a proven remedy for cancer, let alone a 'cancer cure'. There is some evidence, however, that it can be helpful when used in connection with other therapies and it is now prescribed by certain individual practitioners and also used in a number of Dutch, Swiss and German clinics, where its administration is combined with heat treatments – Steiner believed that warmth stimulates the activities of the Ego in the body – and artistic exercises intended to calm and harmonize the emotions.[3]

Iscador is manufactured using extremely complex techniques designed to strengthen the supposed independent and individualistic qualities of the mistletoe by further isolating it from outside forces, such as the earth's spin. No other plant-derived remedy used in anthroposophical medicine is the product of quite such extraordinary processes as those used in the manufacture of Iscador. Yet the preparation of almost all such medicaments demands lengthy and complicated manipulations of not only the plant, the raw material of the medicine, but of the soil on which that plant was grown. For cultivated plants used in anthroposophical medicine are, whenever possible, grown in accordance with the principles of biodynamic agriculture. Some brief descriptions of these are given in Appendix II; here it suffices to say that biodynamic farming and gardening goes beyond ordinary organic husbandry in that, as well as avoiding the use of synthesized fertilizers and pesticides, the biodyamic agriculturalist takes into account cosmic and terrestrial influences.

Biodynamic composting (see Appendix II) is an essential feature of the preparation of 'vegetabilized metals', of which several are included in the anthroposophical pharmacopoeia, amongst them being *aurum per primula* ('gold through prim-rose'), *cuprum per chamomilla* ('copper through camomile'), and *plumbum per aconitum* ('lead through aconite'). The process begins by a naturally occurring metallic ore, a metal, or a metallic salt, being ground into small particles and used to 'salt' an area of organically fertilized soil which is then seeded. At the end of the growing cycle the plants are harvested and subjected to biodynamic composting. In the following spring the compost is applied to the soil which is reseeded. The harvest from this second seeding is again composted and a third generation of plants is grown. These provide the material which is processed into the 'vegetabil-ized metal' remedy.

The object of the vegetabilization process, which was orig-inally suggested by Steiner in the course of his second series of lectures to physicians, is threefold. In the first place it provides an organic equivalent of the dynamization or potentization which supposedly results from the use of the successive succussions or grindings described earlier. Secondly, it is believed that in this way a plant can be used to guide, as it were, a metal to a particular organ or system, such as the nerve-sense or the metabolic-limb. Finally the vegetabilization is believed to help a weakened biosystem to cope with the sometimes overwhelming strength of the metallic forces.

It is also believed that the degree of heating to which a plant substance is submitted does much to establish an affinity with a particular bodily system. In general plants are submitted either to a cold process, maceration, in which no artificial heating is involved, to a warm process, in which they are heated to the temperature of the healthy human body, or to a hot process, in which they are, in a sense, cooked. Each of these three modes of preparation corre-sponds to one of the three principles of salt, sulphur and mercury posited by Paracelsus and the spagyric physicians who succeeded him. Each also has a particular affinity with one of the three bodily systems, the rhythmic, the metabolic-limb and the nerve-sense. The cold process of maceration is an aspect of what Paracelsus termed 'the salt principle' and has an affinity with the nerve-sense system. The warmth process of 'digestion', in which plants are raised to blood temperature, pertains to the 'mercury principle' of Paracelsus and to the rhythmic system, while the 'cooking' processes – infusion and decoction – pertain to 'sulphur' and the meta-bolic-limb system.

Menodoron, a compound plant remedy used in the treatment of menstrual disorders, the ingredients of which include oak bark, marjoram seed, nettle flowers and a type of yarrow commonly known by the name of old man's pepper, provides an example of an anthroposophical medicament which is subjected to the sulphur process in order to tune it to the metabolic system. On the other hand Digestodoron, a compound largely derived from several different varieties of willow and fern and used by anthroposophical physicians in the treatment of all types of rhythmic disturbance of the gastrointestinal tract, from heartburn to constipation and irritable bowel, is given the 'mercury' process of digestion at blood heat. The cold 'salt process' of maceration is applied to such remedies as those derived from aconite and is intended to relieve neuritis and other disorders of the nerve-sense system. Both Menodoron and Digestodoron are members of the group of so-called type remedies which are not intended to be directed against a particular disease but to restore an organ to healthy functioning.

Higher levels of heating than those involved in digestion, infusion and decoction are also employed in the preparation of some anthroposophic remedies. These include distillation, which as explained subsequently is even applied to metals by the use of what is called the mirror process, tostatio, carbonization and cinization.

Tostatio is toasting or roasting, the latter word being used in the same sense as when one talks of roasting coffee beans, rather than in relation to roasting a joint of meat. Tostatio is held to bring out the sulphur aspect ('sulphur' in the same sense as that of Paracelsus) of the substances submitted to it.

Carbonization is the reduction of a plant substance to charcoal by heating it without an adequate supply of air, thus obtaining a product consisting largely of carbon. Anthroposophists consider the properties of this element to indicate its possible use in therapy. They say, for example, that its ability, particularly in the form of charcoal, to absorb gases shows that it has certain connections with the astral body, with the Air system and with the kidneys (it will be remembered that, as mentioned earlier, the renal system is regarded by anthroposophists as relating to Air).

Cinization means reduction to an ash, that is, combustion in the presence of oxygen, with the consequent production of carbon dioxide. In essence this is the same process which is carried out in respiration, and it is held that cinization of a plant provides it with a sort of conductor wire which leads it to the pulmonary region.

Sometimes anthroposophic remedies combine substances derived from both the mineral and vegetable kingdoms. Thus a compound manufactured by the Swiss company WALA for use in cases of muscular rheumatism contains potentized silver and sulphur as well as similarly potentized derivatives of birch and arnica. Another product of the same company is prepared from potentized tin and an extract of bryony roots.

It is not just preparations intended to be supplied and used in accordance with the directions of qualified practitioners in which plant and mineral substances are combined to form a new and unified whole. The popular toothpastes formulated and manufactured by Weleda Ltd on the basis of the principles of anthroposophical pharmacy exhibit the same characteristics. Thus their herbal toothpaste contains such mineral derivatives as potentized silver nitrate and calcium fluoride in combination with herbal extracts and potentized horse-chestnut bark. Similarly the same company's salt toothpaste contains both substances of plant origin, such as the juice of sloes and potentized arum-lily ash, and minerals such as sodium silicate and sodium sulphate.

The fact that some anthroposophical medicines include tin and silver and that, as described earlier, anthroposophical pharmacists devote so much time and effort to the preparation of vegetabilized metals indicates the importance of metals in anthroposophical medical practice. It is believed that the ancient alchemical and astrological tradition that there is a subtle cosmic connection between particular metals and the sun, the moon and the planets – lead and Saturn, iron and Mars, for example – has a certain truth in it. It is also held that some particular organs of the human body have a similar relationship with these cosmic bodies and, through them, link up, as it were, with specific metals. In this way gold links up with the heart through the sun. When potentized metals are therapeutically used in this way, as, in a sense, conveyers of cosmic influences, it is often considered that they should be administered in extremely pure form. This purity is obtained by the use of the mirror process. The metals are sublimated – that is, vapourized and precipitated – as a metallic mirror before being submitted to dynamization and other forms of preparation.

In anthroposophical pharmacy it is not always the case that mineral substances are employed in such highly purified forms as those achieved by the metallic mirror process. Following indications given by Rudolf Steiner, many metallic ores and other minerals are used in their natural state as the raw material for dynamization and other preparatory processes. Such minerals include both naturally occurring ores of metals such as iron, mercury and copper – for example, pyrites, cinnabar and malachite – and minerals which have been imprinted with the life processes of constituents of the animal kingdom. These imprinted processes are believed to differentiate various substances which are more or less chemically identical with one another. For example, chalk, limestone, oystershell and crabstone are all largely made up of calcium carbonate, yet anthroposophical physicians use each of them for different therapeutical purposes, differentiated from one another by the processes which have gone into their disposition or biochemical 'manufacture'. Crabstone has come into existence as a result of a series of depositions and dissolvings in the stomach of the crab, oystershell is the result of a once-and-final deposition of layers of calcium carbonate, while chalk and limestone, although originating from the shells of minute sea creatures, are the product of complex geological processes involving heat and pressure which have taken place over enormously long timespans. The imprints that are embodied in these four different varieties of calcium carbonate, say students of anthroposophical medicine, make them suitable agents for treatments which have many different desired results. Thus oystershell, with its rhythmically built-up growth layers, carries the imprint of the processes which have created it and is used as an ingredient in remedies designed to restore rhythm and order to a disturbed calcium metabolism.

The seemingly 'poetic' – in fact, Imaginative, Inspirational and Intuitive – approach of anthroposophical physicians to possible remedies which is apparent in relationship to mistletoe and the development of Iscador is also discernible in relation to components of the mineral kingdom. Thus iron pyrites, a naturally occurring compound of iron and sulphur, has been considered in this way. *Fundamentals of Therapy*, a book written by Dr Ita Wegman and Rudolf Steiner towards the end of the latter's life, informs us that pyrites could more correctly be termed 'the pyrites process' and that in it, as though frozen over periods of geological time, is all that can result from the cooperation of iron and sulphur.

This cooperation, so it is asserted, makes dynamized pyrites, whether used on its own or in conjunction with other remedial substances, an effective remedy for some types of bronchitis and allied disorders which have their origin at the point where the blood and breathing systems of the mammalian body enter into relationship with one another. The iron-process imprint carried by pyrites is thought to have an especial relationship with the body's system of blood circulation, while the sulphur-process imprint is believed to have a similar relationship with the mediation between breath and blood. If this interaction between breath and blood is not operating properly the iron/sulphur combination can, claimed Rudolf Steiner and Dr Wegman, restore normality and, in a sense, take over the mediation process, the iron-process imprint entering the blood circulation and the imprinted sulphur process passing from the circulatory system to that associated with breathing.

Similarly, the mercury/sulphur processes imprinted upon, and locked or frozen into, cinnabar, a naturally occurring form of mercuric sulphide, are released by dynamization and other preparatory work carried out by anthroposophical pharmacists and used in therapy when the physician believes that at work in an organism are biological functions which have become detached and partially independent of the control of the organism as a whole.

Another metal which, like both iron and mercury, has a certain affinity for sulphur is antimony, widely used in the past by practitioners of Paracelsian medicine. Anthroposophical physicians see antimony as having locked within it the same subtle forces as those which lie behind the complex chemical and biological changes which take place during blood coagulation. In the astral body, so it is said, these forces, similar to those frozen in antimony, work outwards, towards those things exterior to the organism, and dynamized antimony preparations are prescribed for internal use when the anthroposophical physician desires to strengthen those astral centrifugal forces. When some form of antimony, such as an ointment containing that metal, is applied externally, as in certain forms of skin disease believed to have their origins in excessive 'astral centrifugalism', it has precisely the opposite effect. It is as if the centrifugal forces radiating from the antimony outside the organism block and counteract those radiating outwards from the astral body.

Many of the chemical compounds of antimony are harmful to life – for example, tartar emetic, a favourite weapon of the nineteenth-century poisoner. Many of the compounds of mercury, such as cinnabar, are also poisonous, and the same is true of most salts of lead and gold, both used in anthroposophical medicine. Is there any danger, then, in the use of the anthroposophic remedies containing potentized derivatives of mercury, lead and other poisonous heavy metals? Is there, for example, some possibility that the amount of lead in the blood may rise to a dangerous level, producing chronic lead poisoning and possible brain, liver or kidney damage?

While it is, of course, essential that stringent safeguards should protect the public from the dangers associated with heavy-metal poisoning there seems to be no doubt that there is no danger of this sort which could possibly arise from the way in which, for over sixty years, dynamized heavy metals have been used in anthroposophical medical practice. Take, for example, lead. Some of the salts of this metal are so poisonous that they have probably affected the course of history. Examination of the skeletons of citizens of the Roman Empire has shown the presence of lead, probably deliberately used in the form of lead acetate to sweeten sour wine; so high are the levels of lead in these skeletons that it is likely that a very high proportion of imperial citizens suffered from chronic lead poisoning of such intensity that their mental abilities were seriously impaired. It has been seriously suggested that this was at least a contributory factor to the fall of Rome and the Western Empire. However, no such chronic poisoning, or anything even remotely approximate to it, could conceivably be caused by the use of lead and its salts *as they are employed in anthroposophical medicine.*

What the anthroposophical practitioner is concerned with in his use of lead and other metals is not the metal itself, but the subtle strengths of the process imprint which is locked or frozen into it. Thus lead and its salts are only used in high potencies, dynamized by rhythmic successions or triturations, in which very little, if any, of the original metal has survived in the remedy which is administered to the patient by injection or by mouth. It will be remembered that it can be arithmetically calculated that no trace of the molecules of the raw material of any dynamized remedy remains at potencies of 23x and above. This, of course, applies to medicines derived from lead and other heavy metals just as much as to those derived from harmless plant and mineral substances. Even at lower potencies the dynamization is sufficiently high to ensure that the remaining amounts of lead or lead salts are almost infinitesimally small: a simple mathematical calculation shows that in the quite commonly employed twentieth decimal potency a lead-derived remedy would have to be injected into a patient's body at a rate in excess of 1000 tons a day before there was even a remote possibility of inducing lead poisoning at even a subclinical level. The same applies to other heavy metals dynamized to high decimal potencies.

An unusual group of anthroposophic mineral remedies are the compositions[4] which are modelled on the make-up and functioning of particular curative plants. Examples of these are *solutio siliceae* composition and *solutio ferri* composition. The former, employed in anthroposophical medicine as a component of therapies for conditions as seemingly diverse as chronic nephritis and eczema, is modelled on the equisetum plant, commonly known as horsetail, and contains sulphur, flint (which provides the silica) and salts of calcium, potassium and sodium. These substances are not bonded together in the chemical sense of the word but are bound together by a process which can most easily be understood if it is thought of as 'cementing'. The ingredients of *solutio ferri* composition, employed for therapeutic purposes which include the stimulation of all aspects of the activity of the blood, are cemented together in a similar fashion. These include sulphur, sodium and potassium salts, but the ingredient which dominates the composition, modelled on the nettle, is iron.

It is possible to regard these remedies formulated on the models of curative plants as being anthroposophical equivalents of the synthesized products, chemically identical with natural substances, which are widely used in orthodox medicine – for example, the digitalis manufactured from chemical substances as a substitute for that extracted from foxgloves. But in formulating these compositions anthroposophical pharmacists are not attempting to obtain the equivalent of alkaloids or other particular components of plants; instead they are trying to obtain a mineral equivalent of the healing functions of the entire plant.

Another composition of the same group of remedies, although of considerably later origin, is *solutio alkalina*, used as a general therapy in cases of weakness and degeneration and supposedly acting on the human organism in very much the same way as that in which a biodynamic compost acts on a sick and devitalized soil. *Solutio alkalina* has been formulated on principles which recall the old alchemical axiom of *solve et coagula*, 'dissolve and coagulate', and which can be discerned in the mineral, animal and vegetable kingdoms. In the vegetable kingdom seed germination and the dissolution of the seed which accompanies that process represents the *solve* principle, while *coagula* is represented by blossoming and fruiting. The same principles can be discerned, say anthroposophists, in cellular division and the processes of colloid development. *Solutio alkalina* is produced by applying the processes of decomposition and combustion – inorganic equivalents to the *solve* and *coagula* of germination and blossoming – to plant substances, the object of this being to provide a remedy saturated with the imprint of the essential being of the original plants and capable of restoring to harmonious interaction the anabolic and catabolic (building-up and breaking-down) functions of a human organism.

Flint, mentioned above as a constituent of *solutio siliceae* compound, is a naturally occurring mineral which is formed around the remains of fossil sponges. As such it does not consist of pure silica, but contains extraneous material incorporated into the structure of the individual flintstone at the time of its formation. Other natural ores and minerals used in anthroposophical pharmacy also contain what are, from the point of view of the chemist, impurities. Thus all naturally occurring lead and zinc ores contain appreciable amounts of silver, while most pyrites contains some elemental substance other than iron or sulphur.

The presence of such impurities seems to have worried some early students of Rudolf Steiner's teachings concerning medicine and pharmacy. Later on such worries were assuaged by arguments that the supposed impurities supplied the human biosystem with minute amounts of trace elements required for its healthy functioning. This may be true, but it seems unlikely. The trace elements in question are only present in the raw minerals in very small quantities and, by the time the successive rhythmic dilutions of dynamization have been carried out, they cannot be present at all on a chemical level – the level at which trace elements operate physiologically – in the final product. The real rationale for the use of ores and minerals incorporating impurities would seem to be that, as these were incorporated in the host mineral as the result of natural processes which have created that mineral, *they carry part of the process imprint*; without them the full imprint of the frozen process would not be available for unlocking by dynamization procedures.

Cosmic factors – that is to say, the rhythm of the seasons, solar, lunar and planetary influences – are taken into account in the manufacture of all anthroposophic pharmaceuticals.

For example, it is not usual to carry out the succussions involved in dynamization procedures during the two hours following noon; this is because there seems to be some solar influence, an element of a diurnal cycle, which makes succussions and triturations carried out during those hours somewhat less effective in potentizing than is usually the case.

Seasonal changes, correlating with the solar cycle which lasts from one spring equinox to another, are of particular significance in the preparation of remedies derived partially or wholly from the vegetable kingdom. This applies even when the plant substance in question is available, unlike, say, blossoms or berries, at all times of the year. So barks and roots intended to be used in remedies designed to vitalize the anabolic – building-up – functions of the organism, or to counter sclerosis – the ageing and hardening of the organism – are gathered in the spring, when nature is burgeoning. On the other hand, those intended to have a catabolic effect – to produce hardening and consolidation, 'inwardness' – are gathered in the autumn, when plant functions are tending toward the same end.

There is, of course, nothing entirely new in the concern for cosmic factors which is displayed by anthroposophical pharmacists and those who employ the medicaments prepared by them. For centuries, perhaps millennia, a similar concern has been apparent amongst those practising traditional healing arts. Thus practitioners of the ancient system of Ayurvedic medicine have always held that a combination of honey and rose petals which has been rhythmically exposed to sunlight has a quite different effect on the emotional life of those who partake of it than does the same mixture if it has been exposed to moonlight. Similarly, many of those apothecaries and alchemically inclined physicians of the sixteenth and seventeenth centuries who prepared and distilled herbal and mineral elixirs carefully correlated various stages of the work with seasonal influences, while the authors of many alchemical treatises insisted that coagulation, rectification and other laboratory techniques should only be carried out when the seven heavenly 'wanderers' – the sun, the moon, Mercury, Venus, Mars, Jupiter and Saturn

– were in particular alignments with each other, with the moon's nodes, known as the 'Dragon's Head and Tail', and with the twelve constellations of the tropical (moving) zodiac.

In its consideration for cosmic influences anthroposophical medicine and pharmacy are, then, in conformity with ancient traditions and perhaps owe something to them. The same is true, as I have attempted to make apparent in preceding chapters, of many other aspects of such medicine and the theoretical concepts which underlie its practice.

This does not mean, however, that anthroposophical medicine is no more than a codification of old traditions, beliefs and peasant superstitions. It may well be, as is believed by many students of the life and work of Steiner, that these old traditions were the corrupted remnants of the wisdom derived from a primitive, instinctive clairvoyance, the capacity for which no longer exists in men and women of the present day, the times for which it was suited having long passed into history. On this hypothesis the achievement of Rudolf Steiner was to extract the nuggets of gold from the spoil tip of the past and to fuse them with the new 'philosophical gold' which he had derived from the use of the higher faculties, belonging to the future not the past, of Imagination, Inspiration and Intuition.

Whether this was so or not, there can be no doubt that many of the pharmaceutical processes and formulations which have been described in this chapter owe more to indications given by Steiner than to tradition. Through their employment the anthroposophical physician has had made available to him or her a very large number of therapeutic preparations in addition to those which are used in orthodox medicine. It would be possible to use these preparations in a thoroughly empirical and mechanical way – 'for condition y one uses preparation p, q and r',and so on. But the complex theoretical structure, based on spiritual insight, which underlies anthroposophical medicine should ensure that the physician does not fall into this trap but applies his knowledge creatively, always striving, in Steiner's own words, 'to work in accordance with *becoming* nature'.

PART TWO

Rudolf Steiner and the Holistic Approach to Healthy Living

4

Childhood Health and Development

It is now generally accepted that the physical constitution of a young child is to some extent determined by prenatal influences which it undergoes in the embryonic stage. A very large number of chemical substances cross the placental barrier, are incorporated into the physical structure of the embryonic body, and exert an effect, sometimes a lifelong effect, on the constitution of the child. The most publicized examples of such chemical influences on the embryo have, of course, been those children of the 1960s who were born with severe physical deformities because their mothers had taken a supposedly harmless sleeping pill. More recently almost as much attention has been given to the tragic cases of children born with a physical dependence on heroin, their drug-addict mothers having passed heroin through the placenta in sufficient quantities to create an addicted embryo. Apart from such spectacular cases there is some reason to think that many other allegedly harmless chemicals, such as food additives and pesticides which have entered the food chain, may pass from a pregnant woman to the embryo within her, thus exerting a permanent and perhaps harmful influence on the health of the, as yet unborn, child.

This is now taken almost for granted, and many pregnant mothers make some effort to reduce their intake of substances which might be harmful to their children. It was not, however, so widely accepted over sixty years ago when Rudolf Steiner drew attention to the importance of the *quality* of the substances ingested by the mother during pregnancy in relation to the health of her child. At that time the general attitude to pregnancy was a reductionist one, the womb being considered as little more than a protoplasmic incubator/feeding system – feed the mother with plenty of protein, fat and carbohydrates, and all, so it was thought, would be well.

While in the present day the general tenor of Steiner's teachings regarding the causative relationship between the foods and other substances entering the mother's body and the physical condition of the embryo is almost looked upon as a truism, the same does not apply to more particular aspects of those teachings. Thus, for example, he taught that meat and potatoes were best largely avoided by the prospective mother, in so far as it was possible for her to do so, because, so he said, they make the organs of the embryo 'excessively physical', grosser, and thus more difficult for the incarnating Ego to penetrate properly. The pregnant woman, he said, should replace most of her normal intake of meat with proteins derived from milk, such as cottage cheese; she should not, however, be completely veg tarian if she had a genuine longing for animal protein – in Steiner's own words, 'It is better to eat meat than to *think* meat.'[1]

There is an emphasis on the 'natural' not only in anthroposophical medicine but in many other applications of Rudolf Steiner's teachings. Thus anthroposophical architects tend to design buildings incorporating flowing lines reminiscent of plant forms, anthroposophical farmers avoid using artificial fertilizers and synthetic pesticides, and so on. It is thus not surprising that anthroposophical paediatricians have always been enthusiastic advocates of breast feeding, even when the fashion for bottle feeding was at its height. They have pointed out that, in spite of all the efforts made by manufacturers of baby foods to produce a substance duplicating the composition of human mothers' milk, no such exact duplication has been achieved. Nor, it is asserted, is success possible. For even if the fatty acids, enzymes, etc., which are present in human milk could be synthesized, the synthetic product would still not contain the antibodies which have been developed inside the mother's body and which confer protection against infection until such time as her baby's body has been able to manufacture its own antibodies. Furthermore it would be impossible to develop a large enough range of synthetics to duplicate the continual changes in the content of an individual mother's milk, changes which normally ensure that her milk is always suitable for the particular stage of growth at which her child has arrived.

If natural breast feeding of a child is either impossible or has to be supplemented, anthroposophical physicians recommend the use of cows' milk derived from animals fed biodynamically or organically. As this contains much higher amounts of mineral salts and protein than human milk it is usually diluted and sometimes supplemented by additional lactose (milk sugar) in which it is comparatively low. Cows' milk fed in undiluted form is believed to result in an undesirable acceleration of the baby's development.

A similar speeding-up of the developmental process, a sort of infantile premature ageing, is believed to arise from introducing fish, meat and eggs into the child's diet at too early a stage of the weaning process. All such food contains substantial amounts of first-class proteins and is productive of a certain precocity of development (the child's alertness and emotional reactions being noticeable at a very early stage) which is sometimes considered a desirable trait. A few years later, however, this precocity can develop in unwished-for directions, the child becoming excessively restless, active and even aggressive.

A similar effect, so it is believed, can result from initiating weaning at too early an age, and the mother is urged to give her baby an unsupplemented diet of her own milk, supposing the supply to be sufficient, until it reaches the age of five months. In the case of babies whose diet has had to be supplemented with bottle feeds, or who have been entirely bottle fed, it is thought advisable to begin the process a month or so earlier. The baby's first solid food should consist entirely of vegetables – at least one anthroposophical paediatrician considers mashed carrots to be ideal for the purpose – and be given only once a day. After a fortnight or so a second meal, perhaps a purée of apples and ground-up rusks, is given, and from the sixth month a third meal, usually some form of cereals, is added to the daily menu.

Throughout the second six months of life more and more items are added to the child's diet, but still no meat or eggs. Steiner taught that the young child is not really ready to deal with the alien etheric forces present in meat and that to be forced to do so leads to a premature awakening of certain metabolic processes. Eggs, he said, have a somewhat similar effect and can reduce or even destroy the child's natural desire for the foods which are best for it at a particular stage of its development. Rudolf Steiner does, in fact, seem to have been generally suspicious of eggs, as is shown by Franz Kafka's diary note of a lecture he attended in 1911:

The efforts of Dr Steiner will only succeed if the Ahriminian [*sic*] forces do not get the upper hand.

He eats two litres of emulsion of almonds and fruits that grow in the air.

He communicates with his absent disciples by means of thought-forms. . . .

Mrs F.: 'I have a poor memory.' Dr S.: 'Eat no eggs.'[2]

The ideas that a child is not capable of properly digesting meat and eggs at an early age and that the inclusion of such foods in the diet can lead to undesirable results are clearly controversial. There can be no doubt, however, of the truth of Rudolf Steiner's assertion, now confirmed by experimental observation, that the human heat-regulating mechanism which keeps the adult body temperature at a fairly constant 37° C is only partially developed in the young child. As a consequence of this there can be wild fluctuations in the temperature of any baby. Left in a closed car in direct sunlight, its temperature can rise to danger levels within a few minutes; not adequately wrapped up, it can suffer from hypothermia in a physical environment in which adults only need light clothing. Such wrapping-up, say anthroposophical paediatricians, should always be in natural materials – at first wool, later on silk, cotton and linen can also be employed. Even if synthetic substitutes have the same, or better, insulating qualities than natural materials they do not let the skin breathe properly; nor do they embody, so it is said, the cosmic principle of warmth, the word Rudolf Steiner used when referring to what the ancients called the element of Fire.

In view of the great importance anthroposophists attach to keeping babies warm, it may seem rather surprising that they are resolutely hostile to more than a minimum of warm bathing; in particular they are opposed to subjecting a newborn child to a lengthy and elaborate cleansing. This, they claim, not only subjects the baby to a major stress which may produce undesirable and long-lasting psychological effects but removes a natural waxy sheath which helps the child to conserve warmth for the first few days of its life and is then totally absorbed into the body. Bathing, as far as paediatricians who follow Rudolf Steiner are concerned, is a process which should be introduced only gradually into the child's life and even then it should be practised more gently and sparingly than is usually the case. The idea underlying this conservative approach is that, following the shock of birth, the expulsion of the baby from the warmth and safety of its mother's womb, the new-born child must have further shocks reduced to a minimum. It must be given time to adapt itself slowly and gently to its new and harsher environment. Thus, for example, it must not have bright lights shone on it, nor must it be placed in direct sunlight, until days, probably weeks, after its birth.

It is interesting to note that in the 1970s some non-anthroposophical physicians specializing in obstetrics began to express very similar views to those outlined above: it is asserted by such obstetricians that the noise, excessive light and heat, and atmosphere of pain and fright which are surprisingly common in some maternity hospitals can exert a deleterious, and perhaps permanent, influence on the psychological and physical health of babies subjected to them.

The attitude of some anthroposophical physicians towards such infections as measles and chicken pox – what used to be called 'childhood diseases' before modern immunization techniques made them no longer an almost inevitable part of growing up to adolescence and adulthood – is even more unorthodox than their attitude towards bathing and diet.

They agree, of course, with their more conventional colleagues that such infections are intrinsically undesirable, but they also believe that there is a positive as well as a negative aspect to them.

There is no doubt that this idea strikes most parents of young children as so strange as to be almost perverse. Nevertheless, complex arguments in its favour have been put forward by practitioners of anthroposophical medicine, these arguments being derived from, and only comprehensible in terms of, Rudolf Steiner's teachings regarding the nature of both localized inflammation and the abnormally high body temperatures which are a feature of many infectious diseases, such as those particularly associated with childhood and characterized by abrupt changes in temperature. Such changes can result in a quite minor infection sending a child's body temperature to a level which in an adult would suggest a severe or even life-threatening illness. Most parents have had the experience of summoning medical aid when a child has complained of feeling unwell and shown all the signs of high fever, only to find that by the time the doctor arrives the child feels perfectly well and its temperature has reverted to not much, if anything, above normal. While they are not unknown in childhood, 'cold' diseases (as anthroposophical physicians sometimes refer to arthritis, rheumatism, hardening of the arteries and other illnesses not usually accompanied by a rise in general body temperature) are the characteristic afflictions of age rather than youth.

In anthroposophical medical literature the hot diseases are sometimes referred to as 'fevers' or, if more localized, 'inflammations', and the cold diseases as 'scleroses'; these terms refer to a theory concerning a softening/hardening tendency which is thought to exist in human beings of all ages. There are, say anthroposophical physicians, both hardening (sclerotic) and softening (inflammatory) forces at work in the human body, both of them essential to its healthy functioning. Should, however, either of these forces become overactive or underactive the equilibrium between them is destroyed and the human organism, or component parts of it, becomes sclerotic or inflamed.

It is perhaps symptomatic of the indebtedness of anthroposophical medicine to tradition that its practitioners describe inflammation in the same terms as those used by the Roman physicians of almost two thousand years ago. Inflammation, they say, is characterized by *calor* ('heat'), *dolor* ('pain'), *tumor* ('swelling') and *rubor* ('redness'). With this most practitioners of conventional medicine would be inclined to agree, but it is likely that they would look with considerable doubt on the arguments with which anthroposophical physicians assert that these four classic symptoms are related to, respectively, the Ego, the astral body, the etheric body and the physical body.

The first of these correlations is, within the framework of anthroposophical theory, fairly apparent. The Ego, as was said in an earlier chapter, has a correspondence with the elemental Fire of the ancients – to which concept anthroposophists generally apply, following Rudolf Steiner, the word 'warmth' – so the *calor*, heat, of inflammation can be seen as having at least a verbal association with the Ego. The correspondence between *dolor*, pain, and the astral body is almost equally apparent, for pain is in a sense an overconsciousness, an excessive emotion, and thus can be related to the qualities which Steiner attributed to the astral body. Swelling, *tumor*, always involves a gathering of lymph and other body liquids, regarded by anthroposophical physicians as being, to some extent, particular manifestations of elemental Water which, as was explained in chapter 2, is associated by anthroposophists with the etheric body. *Rubor*, redness, is attributed to the physical body because of its cause, the presence of large quantities of red blood corpuscles whose physicality is apparent.

From the point of view of the critic of anthroposophical medicine such reasoning is a mere juggling with words and, using a somewhat different juggling technique, it is possible to make a quite different series of correlations. It could be argued, for example, that as *tumor*, swelling, extends the area of the body it should be attributed to the physical body; or that as the main constituent of blood, the causative factor in *rubor*, is water, the redness of inflammation should be attributed to the etheric body. Most anthroposophical physicians would probably consider any arguments of this sort somewhat futile, and would point out, reasonably enough, that the most important thing about inflammation is that it is a healing process by which the organism, successfully or unsuccessfully, defends itself from external attack. In other words, inflammation is not always an unmitigated evil. It may be productive of discomfort, even acute discomfort, but, unless the physician can attack the cause of an inflammation, to reduce or subdue that same inflammation is to dismantle the patient's own defences. Thus, for example, it is very easy to dispel the inflammation caused by a painful boil by the use of cortisone derivatives, but the results are often disastrous. Just a few days after the swelling and pain have been 'cured' the patient is often afflicted with more boils and the original boil resumes its full virulence, affecting a much larger area of the skin. Such drastic and unwelcome results of cortisone therapy are so often apparent that its use for skin conditions, widespread only a quarter of a century ago, is now largely confined to those in which bacterial attack is not the primary causative factor.

Orthodox medical practitioners are generally in agreement with their anthroposophical colleagues in seeing both localized inflammations and more general fevers as being defensive reactions against the intrusion of alien forces, such as bacteria, into the human biosystem. Indeed, they have sometimes used deliberately induced fevers as a therapy for infections which do not generally produce this defensive reaction; thus before the general introduction of, first, salvarsan and, later, penicillin as treatments for syphilis it was sometimes found an effective procedure, particularly when the disease had reached the central nervous system, to innoculate the patient with malaria, the resultant high body temperature either killing the organisms responsible for syphilis or so greatly weakening them that they became susceptible to the attacks of the patient's defensive forces, such as antibodies and white blood corpuscles.

While there is no great dispute between medical orthodoxy and anthroposophy as to the defensive function of inflammation and fever, there is a considerable difference between them as to what should be regarded as a suitable therapy. In cases where the body has been attacked by bacteria the

orthodox practitioner will almost always employ either antibiotics or chemical drugs such as those belonging to the
sulphonamide group. Unless, however, there is a real danger
to life or the patient is in a very considerable state of
discomfort, the anthroposophical physician will endeavour
to avoid the use of such drastic remedies and instead let the
infection run its course, supporting the body's own defences
by the administration of medicines which have been manufactured in accordance with anthroposophic principles.
There are no hard and fast rules as to what these remedies
should be, for, as it is the patient rather than the disease
which is being treated, what is considered suitable for Mr
A. in a particular situation will be considered to be quite
unsuitable for Miss B. when she is seemingly suffering from
precisely the same inflammatory condition.

Nevertheless, some anthroposophical remedies are fairly
widely employed in such cases, a combination of dynamized
apis (bee venom) and belladonna being the most notable of
these. Interestingly enough, both these medicaments, particularly the first, are employed against inflammation by physicians practising classical homoeopathy. There is, however,
a quite different rationale for their use which provides a
good illustration of the differences of attitude between
anthroposophical medicine and the classical homoeopathy to
which practitioners influenced by Rudolf Steiner are usually
sympathetic.

The basic premise of homoeopathy is not the so-called
'magic of the minimum dose', the use of high-potency medicines, but the principle of 'like cures like' which was
described on p. 11. That is to say, one treats a particular
illness with potentized medicines which, given in large doses,
would produce symptoms similar to or identical with those
generally associated with that illness; thus coffee, which
usually makes sleep more difficult, is given in potentized
form in order to induce sleep. Apis, bee venom, is thus chosen
by homoeopaths as a remedy against inflammation because
in crude unpotentized doses it produces all the symptoms
of inflammation – pain, swelling, redness and heat. Most
anthroposophical physicians are, as was said above,
sympathetic to homoeopathy and, while not totally

committed to the 'like cures like' concept, would consider the symptoms of a bee sting as an indication that apis *might* be usefully employed as an anti-inflammative. They have, however, other reasons, apart from empirical observation and homoeopathic principle, why they so commonly employ apis in cases of both fever and localized inflammation. These reasons are particularly derived from indications given by Rudolf Steiner in the course of a series of lectures he gave to apiarists and others interested in beekeeping.

There is a certain sense, said Steiner, in which the individual bee, whether it is a worker, a drone or even the ruling queen, is not an organism in its own right. It is a constituent element – admittedly a very complex one – of the true organism, the hive as a biological entity. The hive shares many characteristics with the homes of other social insects, such as wasps and ants, but one of its properties seems to be unique. Save in exceptional circumstances its temperature is maintained at a constant level which approximates to the 37°C of the healthy human being. Rudolf Steiner's intuitive faculties induced him to attach significance to this fact. Warmth (i.e. Fire) was for him the element with which the Ego is particularly correlated, just as he believed Water to be correlated with the etheric body; so he taught that the coincidence of temperature between the hive and the individual human being indicates a certain relationship between the latter and the Ego. Another subtle relationship discerned by Steiner was based on the similarity between the regular six-sided cells of which the honeycomb is made up and the hexagonal crystals of various naturally occurring mineral substances. There was, he said, a polarity to be observed in the hive: on the one hand, its constant temperature showed a subtle link with the human spirit, the Ego; on the other hand, the structure of the honeycomb exhibited a relationship with the mineral kingdom.

Anthroposophical medical practitioners see the polarity of the hive as reminiscent of the polarity tendencies of the Ego in the human biosystem – a hardening, mineralizing, sclerotic tendency manifesting itself at the cephalic pole; a softening, warming tendency manifesting itself at the motor-digestive metabolic pole. This has suggested to them therapeutic uses for apis as, in a sense, the dynamized essence of the hive. It introduces into the human body a softening, heating process of the sort associated with the functioning of the Ego in the metabolic-limb system. Putting it in an inevitably oversimplified way, the administration of apis is the substitution of an artificial inflammation, or softening, process for the defensive inflammation which results from the Ego's reaction to infections at the metabolic pole.

As an anti-pyretic, that is, a medicament prescribed in illnesses with symptoms which include fever, anthroposophical physicians customarily administer apis 3x in conjunction with belladonna in the same potentization. Belladonna, deadly nightshade, is a substance which is also sometimes used by homoeopaths on the basis of the principle of 'like cures like'. Given in large doses it is productive of headaches and other symptoms which are similar to those associated with fever. Anthroposophists, however, use it because they see it as a restorative of the balance between the astral and etheric forces at work in the human organism. Belladonna, they point out, is a perennial which exhibits a most unusual annual growth pattern. In the spring it burgeons in shade, an environment not suitable for most plants, and displays vigorous growth until the time at which its dark blue flowers appear. This fast growth, which seems to be maintained or even accelerated when the belladonna plant is competing for light and food with a host of other plant species, is seen by anthroposophists as evidence that extremely powerful and abundant etheric forces have been at work. At the flowering stage, quite suddenly, belladonna almost ceases its growth, an event which anthroposophical pharmacists and physicians see as resulting from astral influences originating outside the plant. As was explained in chapter 2, Rudolf Steiner taught that plants have only physical and etheric vehicles of manifestation. He held, however, that at the flowering stage all plants make a certain contact with the astral world although they do not normally absorb any of the alien astral 'substances'. Belladonna, however, is considered to be one of the plants that does absorb these outside astral forces which affect the plant in two ways, by checking the vigorous etheric forces associated with growth and by manifesting themselves in the physical processes responsible for the plant's production of toxic alkaloids. Belladonna, then, is seen as a physical expression of a process which balances astral and etheric forces and, as such, a suitable medicament to aid a human organism to overcome a certain astral/etheric disequilibrium which is believed to characterize both fever and local inflammations.

As was said earlier, anthroposophical physicians are not rigidly opposed to the use of antibiotics or sulphonamides and similar chemicals and, if they consider the situation warrants it, will employ these instead of, or as a supplement to, anthroposophical remedies. It is held, however, that the use of such orthodox therapies sometimes results in the effects of an illness lingering on for many months after all overt symptoms have ceased. Thus, for example, Dr Victor Bott has claimed that those treated with only anthroposophical remedies tend to have an acute illness which is immediately followed by a period of vigorous regeneration which often leads to the patient feeling in better shape than was the case before the illness. On the other hand, said Dr Bott, those who have been treated with antibiotics do not experience a feeling of renewal and health, but go on for months complaining of debility and a general feeling of ill health.

The belief that fever and inflammation can be followed by physical renewal, a regeneration of the healing forces of the organism, is the rationale for the anthroposophical paediatrician's concept of a positive side to the characteristic diseases of childhood. The breakdown of proteins, which always accompanies fever, is followed, so it is believed, by a period of renewal and growth which helps the child in its natural development. In the words of H. Müller-Eckhard:

A child contracts childhood diseases in order to become healthier. Faced with the tremendous transformations, adaptations, and forming of habits demanded by the adult order, children have to constantly change, learn and practise. It is quite clear that they can do so far better and more quickly with the help of these childhood illnesses.

It is hard for anyone not fully committed to anthroposophical medicine to go along completely with the sentiments expressed in the above quotation. While some of us who suffered attacks of measles, whooping cough or scarlet fever in childhood can remember the sense of health and vigour which followed upon recovery, we can also remember, or at any rate know about, the very heavy infant mortality which resulted from these diseases when they were more widespread than is the case at the present day. It is difficult not to think that a certain regeneration in some children, resulting in a natural development towards healthy adulthood, is hardly an adequate price to pay for the human suffering involved in the very high infant mortality rates from measles and whooping cough prior to the development of effective modern vaccines. On the other hand, it has to be admitted that in a tiny minority of cases the use of such prophylactic vaccines has resulted in extremely harmful side effects.

While Rudolf Steiner always insisted that numbers should not be regarded as having mystic properties in their own right, it is an undoubted fact that polarities, trinities, quaternaries and septenaries feature more in anthroposophical theory, medical or otherwise, than the law of averages might lead one to expect. Thus there is supposedly a polarity between the processes of sclerosis and inflammation, there are three 'systems' in the human organism, there are four cardinal organs and temperaments, while the septenary recurs in a number of contexts, including child development.

Thus anthroposophical paediatricians and educationalists assert that there is a threefold cycle of seven years leading from birth to full adulthood at the age of twenty-one; whatever the legal age of majority may be, it is considered that no human being is fully mature on all levels until that age has been attained. The end of each of these seven-year cycles is marked by what is in effect a further 'birth' following on physical birth. There are, in the chronological order at which they supposedly take place, an etheric birth, an astral birth and a spiritual birth, this latter being the Ego's attainment of the power of acting on purely objective considerations.

Steiner taught that until about a child's seventh birthday its etheric body remains linked to that of its mother, united by an etheric equivalent of the umbilical chord that once united their physical bodies. The etheric birth usually coincides with the onset of the loss of the child's milk teeth. By this time, say anthroposophists, the child has begun to operate through a material body that is genuinely its own, all the physical substances with which it was endowed at birth having been replaced by matter derived from the food and drink it has ingested over the years.

Anthroposophical educationalists believe that until the etheric birth at the age of seven the child has little capacity for true learning. It is, of course, possible to teach a child to read and write, sometimes even to learn mathematics or a classical language, well before that age has been reached, but it is held that this puts an excessive demand on the cephalic pole of the organism, using up forces which should be conserved for a later stage of development, and can be deleterious to both the physical and mental health of the overtaxed child.[3]

The child's attainment of its seventh birthday means that its growth rate begins to slow down markedly, that etheric forces are now released from the metabolic system for service elsewhere, notably at the cephalic pole, where they are responsible for the development of the ability to memorize, and that the astral body begins to play a much larger part in the functioning of the whole organism.

The astral world is very much the plane of the emotions and, as the functions of a child's astral body become more marked, so does that child develop the faculties of empathy and sympathy. As these faculties develop the child is still capable of cruelty, but no longer, if development has been normal, of that mindless — or, rather, emotionless — cruelty which results from a total inability to comprehend that another living being has feelings of its own.

All the emotional feelings which can be felt by human beings regarding one another, regarding other living beings, and even regarding objects and places, can be classified, said Steiner, as being sympathetic or antipathetic, or fluctuating between these two extremes; in the terminology of anthroposophy, the words 'sympathy' and 'antipathy' are given a much wider meaning than in normal colloquial usage. By 'antipathy' is meant all that drives one away from that which is outside oneself; by 'sympathy' is meant all that drives one toward such external realities. Thus all emotions can be seen as tending towards one or other of these polarities. In life only a minority of things (and beings) exterior to oneself belong absolutely to one or other of these emotional poles; thus most people we meet are neither regarded by us with total antipathy, hatred, nor with total sympathy, love. But everyone we meet we have *some* feeling toward, and such feeling tends to fluctuate between the two poles. One day we meet Mr X and find his conversation mildly interesting – in other words our feelings about him tend towards the pole of sympathy; the next time we meet him he tells us at interminable length about the capabilities of his home computer and we get bored – our feelings fluctuate towards the antipathetic pole.

All of us experience such fluctuations of the emotions, but they are experienced more violently, say anthroposophical physicians and educationalists, by children between the ages of seven and fourteen. They are, in a sense, playthings of the rhythmic dance of the astral forces between the two poles of the emotions. One day a particular child is their closest friend, another day the same child is the subject of intense dislike; one week the child is an obsessive reader, the next it wants to spend all its time in hectic outdoor activities. At times sympathy, in the wide anthroposophical sense of the term, for a particular mode of activity becomes virtually an epidemic amongst the juvenile population, and the sale of, for example, skateboards rises to extraordinary heights, leading to increased investment in skateboard manufacturing capacity. By the time this comes into production, of course, the general attitude has swung towards the pole of antipathy: they are considered a bore and the shops are cluttered with unsold skateboards.

The rhythmic fluctuations between sympathy and antipathy are symptomatic of the general behaviour of children aged between seven and fourteen; there is a rhythmic mobility of the limbs and a common wish for the expression of the inner dance of the emotions through music, poetry and the plastic arts. This desire for rhythmic expression, say anthroposophical educationalists, should be met by being made central to the child's schooling during the relevant years – an academic approach to learning must be avoided and music and the arts should be emphasized and even integrated into the teaching of such subjects as history and languages. Anthroposophical physicians claim that during this 'rhythmic septenary' children are less liable to illnesses than they are at an earlier stage of their lives and, if they do become ill, are more capable of throwing off infections. This, they say, is because during this period the body's rhythmic system is working extremely efficiently and, as a consequence of this, is easily able to restore any temporary disequilibrium between the nerve-sense and motor-digestive systems.

At around the age of fourteen the activities of the astral body over the preceding seven years result in the onset of puberty. Sometimes, of course, this takes place much earlier, and sexual maturity in the purely reproductive sense of the phrase is sometimes experienced at a very early age indeed; on the other hand, some children do not reach physical maturity until some months or even years after their fourteenth birthday. Nevertheless, say anthroposophical physicians, whatever the outward physical appearances may be, the phase of puberty, in the sense of the astral body having fully performed certain developmental functions, is reached at around the date of the child's fourteenth birthday. At this stage the child experiences a sort of 'astral birth', that is to say, astral forces which have been previously engaged in expressing themselves as the many physical developments which have taken place over the preceding seven years are now made available for other tasks.

In the long run this astral birth is extremely advantageous to the adolescent, his or her family, teachers and friends. In the short term, however, the results are extremely unfortunate and may reduce those in contact with the child to near despair. For it is held to be the surgings of these, at first largely uncontrolled, astral forces which are responsible for many of the difficulties of adolescence, from general moodiness to bad temper and outright loutishness. If the astral energies are properly channelled in the adolescent boy or girl, they eventually result in a rise in the general level of consciousness, an increased ability to reason, and so on. If, however, there is a failure to reintegrate the forces of the astral body into the organism as a whole, a variety of psychological disturbances, varying in severity from excessive shyness to delinquency and even schizophrenia, can result.

The mildest form of these is typified by the adolescent boy who blushes easily, finds it difficult to take part in conversations, and replies to civil questions with something very like a porcine grunt. A more extreme variant of what is considered to be the same functional problem − a failure of the Ego properly to control astral energies in their relationship to the etheric body − leads to an obsessive concern with the body, particularly with its sexual attributes and desires, which can, so it is said, ultimately result in a variety of psychological disturbances from erotic mania to schizophrenia. Such an excessive penetration of the physical by the astral can happen to both young men and young women but, according to some anthroposophical physicians, it is much more likely to be experienced by the former than the latter. This is because in the normal course of events the astral bodies of males are more deeply incarnated (i.e. more closely united to the physical body) than those of the opposite sex, so an excessive physicalization of astral forces is nearer the normal condition of young men than young women.

Young women are held to be more liable to experiment, as it were, with the astral energies which have been liberated by puberty − to see what effect their emotions, or seeming emotions, have on other people. Such experimentation shows itself in behaviour which is designed to intrigue, provoke and even arouse the sexual feelings of others, not because of any real desire for those feelings to be physically expressed, but because it is amusing to demonstrate an ability to arouse strong emotions in other human beings. All post-pubertal young women have a tendency to behave in such a way, as do some adolescent boys, but as adulthood approaches the flaunting of astral energies for its own sake usually seems less desirable, the astral body is brought under the control of the Ego, and begins to carry out its function of ordering and structuring the etheric forces. Sometimes, however, the astral forces prove beyond the control of the Ego and strange and impulsive behaviour manifests itself, sometimes reaching a stage of dangerous uncontrollability. What is needed is a strengthening of the Ego, particularly in its functioning at the cephalic pole, thus enabling it to penetrate and control the astral body; and, similarly, a strengthening of the upper astral forces as distinct from those particularly involved with the metabolic pole.

The anthroposophical beliefs concerning the post-pubertal development of young men and women which have been summarized in the preceding paragraphs carry the clear implication that the types of adolescent sexual behaviour which were regarded with tolerance in the permissive social climate of twenty years ago are to be looked upon as either pathological or, at any rate, verging on the pathological. This does not mean that anthroposophical physicians and educationalists advocate some sort of revival of the emotionally strangling attitudes towards any expression of physical feeling which typified the social mores of a century ago. It does mean, however, that they are quite as opposed to what they consider to be a premature sexual development of the adolescent as they are to the premature intellectual development which results from the imposition of dryly intellectual teaching methods on children who have not reached the age of fourteen. Just as in the latter case the diversion of etheric forces from their task of building up the organism may result in the development of a pale and listless child, alienated from his environment and unable to fully enjoy the company of contemporaries educated in ways more hamonious with nature, so in the latter case the diversion of astral energies, which should rightly be used in the development of the ability to think, to the reproductive organs and expressions of physical sexuality results in a stunted growth of the mind. This does not mean that such stunted individuals necessarily give the impression that they are obtuse or even of slightly below average intelligence. On the contrary, they often seem highly intelligent although, perhaps, lacking a capacity for sustained intellectual effort, and some of them are academic high achievers. In the latter cases it is believed that karmic factors are often involved in the premature sexual development and that academic success has been attained in spite of, not because of, the diversion of astral energies into the sexual life. In general, so it is argued, however great the mental development of young men or women who also live intensely active sexual lives, their capacity for creative thought would be still greater if there had not been such early sexual experimentation and fulfilment.

Anthroposophical physicians and paediatricians assert that it is often possible to use therapies which help restore a proper flow of the astral energies in the young. One such therapy is curative eurhythmy, the use of which is not confined to the young but can be relevant to those of any age and, as will be described in a later chapter, is a component element in the holistic treatment of a whole range of disorders. Eurhythmy has some similarity to, but is by no means identical with, eurhythmics (a system of rhythmic body movements which is neither quite dance nor gymnastics, devised by E. Jaques-Dalcroze, 1865–1950). Eurhythmy was devised by Rudolf Steiner, whose second wife, Marie von Sivers Steiner, was a notable exponent of this new mode of bodily expression which is not only a therapy, but an art form in its own right, demanding of skilled performers the harmonious employment and interaction of all the component elements of the human organism, body, soul and spirit or – in Steiner's own terminology – physical/etheric complex, astral body and Ego.

The nature of eurhythmy is undoubtedly more easily understood by witnessing a performance of it than by reading a description of either such a performance or of the principles on which it is based. Very broadly, however, it can be said that anthroposophical eurhythmy is an expression in movement of the essential content of music or literature. It is, in a sense, *visible* music or speech and, as such, is not an art form in which improvisation is appropriate, for the movements are in no sense arbitrary. The performer can no more legitimately substitute one movement for another than a Shakespearean actor can substitute one line for another or an organist can substitute one bar of a Bach fugue for another.

It is not really possible to consider eurhythmy as a dance form, for in all dance, whether it be classical ballet or the *macumba* of Brazilian spiritualism, the stately pavane of sixteenth-century Spain or the rock and roll of the 1960s, the movements of the dancer's trunk are of major importance. In eurhythmy, however, the most essential element in the performer's expertise is the movement of the arms and hands. When witnessing an actual performance it is of these fluid and graceful arm movements that the observer is usually most conscious, even more so than of the music which is being played or of the words, usually poetry but sometimes prose, that are being recited. One's awareness of the existence of the trunks of the performers remains on the very fringe of consciousness. In the case of women eurhythmists, their bodies are, in any case, largely hidden by flowing dresses.

Eurhythmy at its highest, say exponents of the art, goes far beyond the mere expression in movement of the sound of music, song or speech. It is a reflection in movement, as it were, of the great cosmic dance of creation, the activities of the Logos, the Word, of the opening verses of the Gospel according to Saint John. As such, every one of its movements arises, in a sense, from the nature of the abundantly healthy man or woman, for health is always, in the final analysis, an expression in the human organism of the rhythmic harmony of the cosmos. What is more, eurhythmy, being an expression of the ultimate ground of all being, speaks directly to the spirit in all of us – it does not demand the almost mathematical intellectual analysis which is required for the fullest possible appreciation of, say, a Bach fugue or a Lassus motet.

From eurhythmy proper, that is, as both an art form and as an expression of the cosmic dance of harmonious rhythm, are derived both educational and therapeutic eurhythmy. The former, which is used in all Steiner schools, is seen as an important part of the education of the child. Ordinary gymnastics, which are also a part of the curriculum, are seen as developing the dynamic and, to some extent, the static functions of the body – mobility, agility, balance and so on. Eurhythmy is regarded as expressing the essentially similar functions of the entire organism on all its levels: physical, etheric, astral and spiritual.

In curative eurhythmy the movements and gestures of the art form are modified in such a way that they react upon the sick body or the disordered mind. The outward gestures carry inward, it is taught, a harmonizing process which influences the diseased organ or the diseased functioning of the etheric or astral body. It must be remembered that anthroposophical physicians regard all illness, whatever may be its immediate source, such as bacterial invasion, as ultimately resulting from disharmony, lack of equilibrium; consequently the aim of all therapy, whether involving the use of physical medicaments administered orally or by injection, or 'psychic medicaments' such as eurhythmy, is the restoration of equilibrium in the organism and its functioning. If such an equilibrium can be restored and maintained, the organism cannot, by definition, be unwell – the body is subject, of course, to the wear and tear of life and the sclerotic processes which must always accompany ageing, but there is no need, anthroposophical physicians aver, for such normal wear, tear and 'hardening' to result in a state of ill health.

In dealing with the difficulties sometimes experienced by adolescents in coping with the astral energies which are liberated at around the fourteenth birthday, eurhythmy is often complemented by, and integrated with, the employment of a therapeutic mode of a particular type of declamation or speech formation which has been developed by anthroposophists on the basis of indications given by Rudolf Steiner. A detailed description of this is outside the scope of this book, and it suffices to say that each of the four temperaments (which were briefly described in chapter 2 in relation to the cardinal organs) is held to correlate with specific vowel sounds and that certain vowels and consonants are held to have a particular relationship with, respectively, planetary and zodiacal forces.

Physical remedies, usually dynamized anthroposophical medicines, are sometimes prescribed for supposed astral disturbances in both child and adult patients. The exact nature of which particular medicaments are used in therapy will vary from patient to patient, for there is no anthroposophical cook book laying down hard and fast rules which are applied to every case, but a remedy which might be used is a naturally occurring combination of iron, copper and arsenic[4] – 'to give arsenic', said Steiner, 'is to astralize'.

A large proportion of adolescents suffer from skin complaints, and while no one ever died from juvenile acne it is a condition which can cause great mental distress to those who suffer from it. This distress sometimes leads to depression, attacks of acute anxiety and other psychological disturbances. The general attitude of anthroposophical physicians to juvenile acne provides a good example of a holistic approach. The affliction is seen not so much as a disease of the skin, of real interest only to the dermatologist, but as a symptom of lack of equilibrium, probably involving the astral body, of the organism as a whole. Treatment is therefore primarily directed at restoring harmony – healthy functioning – in all its aspects rather than concentrating on the morbid skin condition. That, it is believed, will eventually clear up if the general health is good. Some anthroposophical physicians believe that the former is more easily achieved if the adolescent acne sufferer is put on a special diet which includes no animal fats whatsoever.

Such a diet sometimes begins with a week or so in which no solid food save fresh apples is eaten. This is followed by two or three months of an exclusively vegetarian diet; at the end of this period the diet, as it contains no meats carrying substantial amounts of fat, remains very largely vegetarian. This type of diet is sometimes supplemented by the administration of dynamized remedies – typically derived from quartz and varieties of seashell – and by the application of hot compresses to which an extract of calendula (marigolds) has been added. A teaspoonful or two of the same extract is usually added to the sufferer's bathwater. Calendula is, in fact, a common ingredient of many anthroposophical skin lotions, ointments and beauty preparations. It is safe, mild, seems to be generally beneficial in its effects, and in more than one British maternity hospital a calendula preparation manufactured by an anthroposophical pharmaceutical company is the only substance, save soap and water, which is applied to babies' skin.

Juvenile acne *can* continue into later life and become associated with a number of other skin conditions, in which case it may be an expression of an underlying disequilibrium, the causes of which are more deeply rooted than those associated with the skin disorders of the adolescent. In general, however, provided the all-round health is good, all traces of juvenile acne should be fast disappearing by the age of twenty-one, the time at which the young man or woman goes though his or her fourth 'birth' – the attainment of a state in which the Ego is fully incarnated and free to develop in the world of the spirit.

5

Healthy Maturity

The seven-year periods which are believed particularly to characterize childhood do not cease with the 'birth' of the Ego but continue throughout maturity and old age. They are not, however, marked by such fundamental changes as those which culminate in the etheric, astral and spiritual births. Very broadly, the significance of each seven-year cycle steadily diminishes with age. It is worth noting, however, that Rudolf Steiner taught that by the age of twenty-eight human beings have developed as far as they can on the basis of the intrinsic developmental qualities with which they are endowed at birth. After this men and women have to rely on what they make of themselves: they either develop further as a result of their own inner strivings or stay 'frozen' spiritually at the level they reached at their twenty-eighth birthday. In certain comparatively rare conditions they lose part of that which they have developed on the basis of their natural endowments, and regress to an earlier stage. Such regression has always existed and has usually resulted from an individual making a conscious choice to follow the path of spiritual regression rather than that of progression; according to at least one anthroposophical practitioner, it is a somewhat more common condition than used to be the case because such a regression can be induced by an addiction to hard drugs.

In a sense, to remain in the 'frozen' state is as unnatural as to regress. As is explained in a later chapter in connection with Rudolf Steiner's cosmogony and its relationship with his extension of the healing art, it is considered that progression is the natural state of humanity, a reflection of cosmic processes of evolution and involution. Progression, of course, in the sense of *spiritual* progression, which is not necessarily accompanied by increasing technological sophistication, which can exist, as Steiner pointed out in his interpretation of certain historical epochs, alongside a spiritual regression, a concern with the manipulation of dense matter as an end in itself.[1]

'Live the life and you will understand the doctrine' is a proverbial expression in some monastic orders and, while anthroposophists do not assert that a particular mode of living will automatically bring about a desirable spiritual progression, they do believe that the right physical, intellectual, and emotional environment, a healthy way of life on all levels of being, will facilitate an individual development which continues through maturity and old age. 'On all levels of being' must be understood quite literally. The anthroposophical physician believes that it is possible to have a sound constitution and to follow a way of life which is in accordance with all the recommendations of nutritionists, specialists in environmental diseases and so on, and still be deeply unhealthy. Even, it is said, if one avoids indulgences of all sorts and eats only wholefoods which are in exactly the right proportions to one another and contain the optimum amounts of minerals and vitamins, it is possible to be suffering from starvation, from a spiritual and/or emotional malnutrition, an inner dryness and debility which no food or drink can alleviate or cure. *Mann ist was der isst* ('man is what he eats') is an old German pun and, in a sense, the anthroposophist is in complete agreement with it. For he or she feels that what is physically eaten is only part of one's daily diet: what one reads, watches or listens to is also 'food', and in some ways a more important part of one's diet than material food and drink.

This does not mean that either anthroposophists in general, or medical practitioners who have been influenced by Rudolf Steiner's teachings in particular, advocate the disregard for the physical body and its environment which has characterized certain ascetic sects, mostly of oriental origin. Spirit redeems matter, said Steiner, and those who follow him believe that at the present time the spiritual development of humanity involves the incarnation of the Ego in astral, etheric and physical bodies. In other words, the body is the temple which not only *contains* the spirit but has every atom of its structure saturated *with* the spirit. The body, as the temple of the spirit, must not be desecrated by abusing it by, for example, eating devitalized foods, indulging in addictive drugs or bombarding it with more sense impressions than it can handle.

Such an attitude – that keeping one's bodily organism in health is not only advisable but a positive duty – necessarily involves adopting a lifestyle rather different from that which is the norm in contemporary urban society. Take, for example, the anthroposophical assertion that one must carefully regulate the extent of the organism's subjection to sense impressions, as all such exterior stimuli result in certain breaking-down, or catabolic, processes in the individual. Throughout the waking life of the individual, say anthroposophical physicians, the catabolic processes are dominant in the organism and the anabolic, building-up, processes are quiescent. During normal sleep the position is reversed, and throughout the hours of the night the essentially anabolic process of regeneration of the nerve-sense system takes place.

Catabolic dominance is inseparable from full consciousness – thought and the processes involved in the perception and analysis of the impressions received through the senses cannot be properly carried out if the subtle energies available to the organism as a whole are being largely employed in the regeneration and renewal of the nerve-sense system. This implies that thinking, processing sense impressions and everything which is involved in ordinary life when we are not actually asleep are literally exhausting – we use up, as it were, elements of the nerve-sense system just as an electric fire uses up electricity when it is switched on.

If the demands made upon the nerve-sense system are too great, it tends to suffer damage and, eventually, such damage may reach a stage at which it is virtually irreparable. Such excessive demands can be made by the normal processes of living in an industrialized urban society, simply by surrendering oneself to the sensory stimuli that clamour for attention. Thus, as has been pointed out by Dr Walter Buhler, if one simultaneously eats a meal, reads a newspaper and half listens to the radio, one is, without fully realizing it, subjecting one's nerve-sense system to a flood of sense impressions involving taste, hearing and sight. This is simply asking too much of the system and leads to an undesirable dissipation of energies. Because one is doing three things at once, none of the sense impressions received are processed as fully as they should be – food is not fully tasted, the music on the radio is not fully heard and appreciated and elements of the newspaper story which is being read are not properly understood.

Almost all of us in the Western world feel that 'there aren't enough hours in the day', regularly try to do two or three things at the same time in exactly the way Dr Buhler has described, and feel that there is no great harm in it. According to anthroposophical physicians, however, by adopting such a lifestyle we are in danger of damaging our nerve-sense systems in very much the same way as we would damage our digestive systems if we felt that social pressures necessitated our eating eight large meals a day. Just as subjecting our stomachs to such an excessive food intake would undoubtedly result in bodily illness, at best violent indigestion, so an excessive intake of sensory impressions inevitably results in what is most easily thought of as an illness of the soul, a sort of 'psychic indigestion'. The mind is, so to speak, crammed with undigested experiences – the sufferer feels 'under stress', 'anxious' or 'wound up'. Eventually the alien, undigested, experiences in the mind may produce effects analogous to those which are believed to result from alien, undigested proteins in the body – that is to say, they manifest themselves physically, the individual concerned feeling tense and unwell or even developing specific physical complaints.

Illnesses which result from sensory overstimulation are by far the commonest physical complaints affecting mature human beings in the Western world. They include diseases affecting the digestive system, gastric and duodenal ulcers being the most notable of these, the heart and circulatory system, kidneys, lungs and, particularly in women, the organs of reproduction. At one time the most common of these stress-induced conditions were gastric and duodenal ulcers, but at the present time hypertension, that is, raised blood pressure, is perhaps the most widespread, affecting a sizeable proportion of the adult population and seemingly becoming more frequent amongst both men and women. High blood pressure, claim anthroposophical physicians, can result not only from a hardening and narrowing of the arteries, but from a stress-induced failure of the will and a consequent loss of muscle tone which affects the entire circulatory system.

To grasp this idea it has to be remembered that Rudolf Steiner taught that the will pertained to the metabolic system and not, as might be at first thought, to the nerve-sense system. If energies which should properly be employed in the metabolic system are, in fact, engaged in the nerve-sense system in desperately attempting to 'digest' the flood of sense impressions to which the organism is subjected by its environment, then the metabolic will-to-life will inevitably suffer. In a sense it is as though the man or woman whose nerve-sense processes make demands on the energies which should be available to the metabolic system in general, and the will in particular, is not fully incarnated (i.e. as though the Ego was not properly interacting with the astral, etheric and physical bodies). In such individuals there is a lack of muscle tone which betrays itself in the general carriage and appearance; more basic than the lack of will in the visible musculature is that which exists in those muscles which are not directly visible, of which the most important is the heart itself.

Such a condition can eventually reach a stage at which more or less the same possibilities exist as those associated with the classic scleroses and arterial narrowing generally referred to as hardening of the arteries. That is to say, the blood supply to the heart muscle may become so restricted that angina results, or the small clots which continually form in the bloodstream and are normally dispersed by the action of the white corpuscles and other components of the body's defensive system block a narrowed artery before the dispersal can be effected. At its worst this results in a myocardial infarction, the heart attack of everyday speech.

That this condition is largely a result of stress, an overloading of the nerve-sense system by making too great demands upon it, seems highly probable. In this connection it is interesting to note that post-mortem examinations carried out on American soldiers killed in Korea, the average age of these casualties being only just over twenty-two years, showed that over threequarters of them exhibited the first symptoms of coronary heart disease, undoubtedly resulting largely from the stress of battle. This is not to say, of course, that the high consumption of animal fats in the USA did not play some causative part in these young men's condition, but it is interesting to note that amongst members of contemplative monastic orders in both Europe and North America myocardial infarction is rare. This applies whether or not the dietary regimen of a particular order does or does not include animal fats.

In treating cardiac infarction the anthroposophical physician always bears in mind that the therapy administered can be little more than palliative unless the patient is prepared to change his or her way of life. Such a change is usually initiated by a period of absolute rest and quiet, following which the patient must devote much of the attention he or she previously gave to, say, building up a business or being a company's best salesman to spiritual matters – 'spiritual' in the anthroposophical sense, of course, applies to art, music, poetry and so on, as well as the prayer and contemplation which are part of ordinary religious life.

In the treatment which leads up to such a change in lifestyle, and which may have to be continued until long after the change has fully taken effect, there are available to the anthroposophical physician not only the drugs which are used in ordinary medicine, such as anticoagulants, but a number of specifically anthroposophical remedies, such as Cardiodoron, compounded in accordance with an indication given by Rudolf Steiner, and 'gold through primrose', one of the naturally dynamized vegetabilized metals. Other anthroposophical medicaments that might be prescribed include a 3x-potentized extract of the strophantus seed, gold in the thirtieth decimal potency (at which stage of dynamization none of the original material remains but only the imprint of the gold process), and a 3x derivative of the sloe, the fruit of the blackthorn.

All the above remedial preparations, save Cardiodoron, which is applicable to all disorders of the heart, are normally only employed in circumstances in which heart disease has had its origin in a disequilibrium resulting from an excessive call having been made on the nerve-sense pole. In circumstances in which the disequilibrium is of a converse nature, having arisen as a result of too great demands having been made upon the forces available at the metabolic pole, a quite different range of anthroposophical remedies might be employed by the physician. Thus in such 'soft' diseases of the heart as myocarditis and pericarditis the anthroposophical physician might administer medicines including silver 30x, a potentized combination of tin and bryonia, and dynamized gold, the latter being given in a comparatively low potency rather than the very high potencies in which the metal – or, rather, the metallic process – is usually prescribed for 'hard' disorders.

In a sense anthroposophists see the aetiology of all diseases as being concerned with an inner disharmony of function and disequilibrium of force. It is not only life-threatening disorders such as diseases of the heart which are believed to result from disharmony. An essentially similar inner disequilibrium can lead to chronic conditions which, while they are not life-threatening, can adversely affect the quality of life. Notable amongst these are a variety of skin complaints ranging from mild dandruff, which is not really a hair condition but a skin disorder associated with a certain strain of yeast, to disfiguring and distressing weeping eczema.

The skin is, of course, primarily an organ of sensation, the outer covering through which we experience the sense of touch. As such it pertains particularly to the nerve-sense system, to the domain of the cephalic pole, a classification which is confirmed, say anthroposophical physicians, by its function as the 'form shaper' of the body which it enfolds. There is in the healthy human skin a certain harmonization of two opposite but essential functions, the centripetal inward-flowing astral forces whose tendency is to a concentration of form and the centrifugal etheric forces which, without the counteracting astral influences, would result in shapeless growth and unrestrained cell proliferation. These forces are never in total balance: at any given time one of them predominates, although in a healthy human being not to the point at which pathological changes become apparent.

In a child, particularly a young child, it is the etheric forces which are dominant, as was explained in the preceding chapter. This sometimes results in a growth rate which parents find almost alarming – the child is said to be 'shooting up', bursting out of its clothes or even 'outgrowing its strength' – but which usually slows down in the mid-teens as the abounding etheric currents are gradually but steadily brought under the control of the astral body. In old age, on the other hand, it is the astral, centripetal forces which are predominant and, in extreme old age a certain desiccation amounting to virtual shrinkage becomes notice-able. There is nothing undesirable about this so long as the etheric forces remain sufficiently active to carry out their proper functions in old age, that is, coping with the demands made upon them by the organism as a whole, carrying out the essential processes of renewal which should follow upon some accidental damage from, for example, a scald, a cut or a bruise, and so on. Provided the etheric forces remain adequate for such purposes their waning and the slowly increasing predominance of the centripetal astral forces is in no way pathological but is a natural and desirable prep-aration for death and the period of spiritual rest which follows and enables the Ego to make itself ready for its next incarnation.

In the mature human being, that is to say, the young or middle-aged adult, the two processes are in a rough equilib-rium; there is no longer the etheric vitality which ensures that a graze or cut suffered by a child heals with extraordi-nary rapidity, but neither is there the very slow regeneration which follows upon similar damage to an elderly body. When such an adult suffers from a chronic skin complaint it is usually, say anthroposophists, an indication of what is an undue disequilibrium between the polarized forces for the patient's age – in other words, a disequilibrium which is normal at eight or eighty years old might well result in skin disorders if it takes place in the body of a forty year old man or woman.

It is possible to consider the same phenomenon in relation to, on the one hand, the cephalic pole and the nerve-sense system and, on the other hand, the metabolic pole and the motor-digestive system.

As was said earlier, the skin is primarily a nerve-sense organ, that of touch, and pertains to the cephalic pole. But the polarity of the entire organism extends to each of its constituent organs and elements. Thus the fingers and toes, which clearly pertain to the metabolic-limb, or motor-digestive, system are extremely rich in nerve endings and, as a consequence, in part pertain to the cerebral pole and the nerve-sense system. Obversely the tongue, with which we taste things, is primarily an organ of the nerve-sense system, but its close relationship with the salivary glands, the product of which plays an important part in the preparation of food for digestion, establishes a connection with the metabolic pole and the motor-digestive system. In the case of the skin there are certain of its functions and attributes which suggest both the metabolic pole and the rhythmic system.

The outer layer of the skin, which in normal circumstances consists entirely of dead cells in process of being shed, has a somewhat mineral-like appearance, vaguely reminiscent of mica and some other natural substances. Such a resemblance to mineral 'deadness' rather than to plant-like proliferation is, in fact, a characteristic of the nerve-sense system – a healthy nerve cell seems shrivelled, dying, tending towards the mineral kingdom when its appearance is compared with that of, for example, the spherical form of a healthy red blood cell. Below the outer layer of the skin comes the vascular layer, richly supplied with tiny arterial blood vessels and thus pertaining to the rhythmic system. It is the contractions of these vessels which makes us turn 'pale with fright'; it is their sudden expansion which makes us 'flush with anger' or 'blush with embarrassment'. Thus they convey our emotions, an aspect of our astral life, to those we encounter. Deeper still beneath the horny outer layer of the skin are to be found the hair follicles and the glands which produce sweat and sebum. All these are manifestations of the metabolic pole of the organism, of the centre concerned with growth and renewal.

Many skin disorders can be categorized as relating either to an excessive development of the motor-digestive, metabolic, aspects of skin functions or to an equally excessive development of its nerve-sense, mineralizing aspects. Thus such 'wet' skin disorders as those associated with the formation of pus, weeping eczema and so on can be classified as being related to the metabolic functions, while such 'dry' complaints as ichthyosis and psoriasis can be considered as pertaining more to the nerve-sense system. The former group of complaints are more common amongst young people, in whom the metabolic processes are more active; the latter are more frequently observed amongst the middle-aged and elderly. This is in no sense a hard and fast rule: on occasion wet eczema afflicts the very elderly patient, while ichthyosis, a disease in which the skin becomes thick, roughened and scaly, has been observed in very young children. Nor are all skin diseases capable of being classified into one category or the other. As the anthroposophical physician Victor Bott has pointed out, urticaria – nettle rash – exhibits symptoms which pertain to both the metabolic and nerve-sense systems, for the eruption of watery, tiny blisters suggests a morbid metabolic process, while the intolerable desire to scratch which is almost always associated with the complaint suggests a nerve-sense disorder. In fact, suggests Dr Bott, the presence of the two symptoms at the same time may indicate some malfunctioning of the rhythmic system which, as explained in chapter 2, is believed to harmonize the cephalic and metabolic polarities. A similar aetiology has been suggested by anthroposophical physicians for diseases such as athlete's foot, of which the immediate cause is a fungal infection.

A large number of ointments are used in the practice of anthroposophical medicine but, curiously enough, few of them are regularly employed in the treatment of skin conditions. Thus, in dealing with fungal infections of the type mentioned in the preceding paragraph, the only ointment frequently used is one containing very small quantities of nicotine and copper. This is applied at night after the taking of a very hot bath – heat is believed to strengthen the Ego's capacity to induce effects upon the physical body – to which some calendula (marigold) extract has been added. A similar bath is taken in the morning, but the ointment which is applied each night is replaced by a powder, compounded on the basis of indications given by Rudolf Steiner, the ingredients of which include antimony, silica, arnica and, again, calendula – almost ubiquitous in anthroposophical therapies for dermatological conditions. No ordinary soap must be used in taking the morning and evening baths, nor, indeed, must it be applied at any time to the areas affected by fungal attack. This is because all commonly available toilet soap is alkaline, and an alkaline environment is extremely favourable to the growth of most fungi. Acid is as unfavourable to many yeast and fungal growths as alkali is favourable – a common home remedy for the yeast infections collectively known as thrush is an application of yoghourt or some other variety of sour milk – and anthroposophical physicians recommend the addition of a little vinegar or lemon juice to the water in which the clothes of the sufferers from athlete's foot and similar diseases are rinsed after washing. This serves to neutralize residual alkalinity derived from soap powders and synthetic detergents.

For psoriasis a diet similar to that recommended for juvenile acne (see p. 106) is often prescribed, as are potentized derivatives of fly agaric – the red and white toadstool which, taken in large quantities, has hallucinogenic qualities – and quartz. Various derivatives of the birch tree are also very often administered to the patient suffering from psoriasis and many other skin complaints. Extracts of various parts of this tree are, in fact, in standard usage in anthroposophical medicine and are so popular as a home remedy amongst those who accept Steiner's teachings that some anthroposophists take a course of birch elixir as a spring tonic. Not surprisingly, the anthroposophical enthusiasm for birch is directly derived from Steiner, who in one of the lectures he gave to physicians in 1920 devoted much attention to this tree, in which he discerned many remarkable properties.

Steiner began by pointing out a certain interaction 'between heaven and earth', which exists between the mineral world and the world of the spirit as represented by the human Ego and which takes place in the human body. Men and women, he taught, absorb minerals in their food and drink but the healthy human body does not become 'mineralized' because, in a sense, the mineral forces are crushed and controlled by the Ego. The elimination of salt and other minerals through skin perspiration provides, considered Steiner, an important example of the demineralizing powers of the Ego. At the same time as the human body is demineralizing itself it is 'proteinizing' itself by the transformation of the constituent elements of foreign proteins into its own substance.

Rudolf Steiner discerned a somewhat similar duality of process in the life of the birch. On the one hand, there is the concentration of vegetable proteins in the young leaves of the birch, the enfoldment of which in the spring he saw as a 'vegetable reflection' of the processes at work in young human beings; on the other, there is a demineralization process – analogous to that which takes place at the level of the skin in man and woman – which results in the bark of the tree containing comparatively high concentrations of potassium salts. These contrasting processes, say anthroposophical physicians, bear a certain resemblance to those polarized functions of the human body which, if they become morbidly excessive, manifest themselves as inflammation and sclerosis.

The functional polarity between bark and young leaf, said Steiner, manifests itself in all trees, but is most marked in the birch. As a consequence of this it is held that remedies derived from birch bark, which so efficiently carries out a vegetable demineralizing process, are often effective against the sclerotic, hardening, processes which, at the level of the skin, manifest as dry dermatoses such as psoriasis. Conversely remedies derived from the young leaves of the tree may be prescribed as part of a therapeutic complex used for the treatment of wet skin complaints such as weeping eczema. Once again it must be emphasized that there are no hard and fast rules in anthroposophical medicine, that the physician who diagnoses and prescribes in conformity with the teachings of Rudolf Steiner is concerned, above all, with the application of a methodology based on Imagination,

Inspiration and Intuition for the alleviation and cure of the afflictions of individual human beings. Such an approach necessarily involves the practitioner in prescribing a therapy which he considers suitable to the individual patient, not in mechanically choosing a particular remedy which some reference book indicates as appropriate to a specific physical condition. Therefore birch-bark extracts are not invariably administered to sufferers from sclerotic, dry skin dermatoses, or leaf extracts to those patients who have wet skin disorders. It might on occasion even be considered best to administer these, at first sight self-cancelling, remedies in combination – perhaps an elixir of birch bark as an antisclerotic and a leaf preparation for some other purpose, for example, as a diuretic.

Polarity concepts are clearly of enormous importance in the theoretical structure of anthroposophical medicine, as is instanced by Steiner's teachings concerning the contrasting functions of the metabolic and cephalic poles, the processes of inflammation and sclerosis, and so on. Another polarity, said Steiner, exists between the skin and the liver. Thus the skin has a highly structured appearance with a hard, dry, mineral-like outer layer, while the liver is by contrast shapeless, soft and wet. Again, the blood contained in the liver is largely venous in nature, while that contained in the vascular layer of the skin is largely arterial. Finally, the liver is primarily a metabolic organ, part of the metabolic-limb (motor-digestive) system, while the skin's predominant characteristic relates, as was said on p. 117, to the nerve-sense system. In spite of this polarity the skin and the liver have one very strong resemblance to one another: both have great capacity for cellular regeneration, both are in continual process of renewal. Largely for this reason, said Rudolf Steiner, in some circumstances the skin endeavours to perform functions which properly pertain to the liver which, because of some defect, is temporarily incapable of fully carrying out all of its metabolic functions.

In such cases the polarity which should properly exist between the two organs is diminished and the skin begins to display some of the characteristics of the liver: in outward appearance it loses its 'cold and dry' form and tends towards the warmth and wetness of the liver; its form is no longer so structured and its tactile sensitivity, which relates to the nerve-sense system, becomes reduced, and so on. In skin complaints arising from such a loss of polarity, say anthroposophical physicians, no satisfactory results can be expected unless treatment is directed towards a restoration of normal liver functioning.

Liver complaints are rare in children but, according to anthroposophical practitioners, are more common amongst adults than is generally recognized. The liver, it will be remembered, is one of the four cardinal organs and is attributed to elemental Water, of which almost all fluids are particular aspects. If the liver does not properly control and regulate the body's water this can, so it is held, appear as watery exudations, not only on the skin but elsewhere in the body, which can serve as foci for infection and inflammation.

Rudolf Steiner gave a great deal of attention to providing his medical pupils with detailed indications for the treatment of liver complaints and particularly recommended three medicaments, namely tin, Hepatodoron and Choleodoron. The first of these is usually prescribed as a vegetabilized mineral of the type whose preparation was described on p. 71. The other two are extracted from herbal mixtures compounded on the basis of specific suggestions made by Steiner, the first containing vine leaves and wild strawberry leaves, the second consisting of turmeric and the leaves of the greater celandine. In the choice of these ingredients Steiner presumably employed his intuitive faculties, but it is interesting to note that the choice seems to have been confirmed by the ancient doctrine of signatures which was described on p. 67. Thus the juice of the greater celandine has an appearance vaguely suggestive of bile, turmeric is of a similarly appropriate colour, and so on.

Hepatodoron is believed to have a generally beneficial effect on liver functioning, so it can be prescribed for almost any liver disorder or, indeed, for any variety of complaint, such as some dermatoses, which are considered to originate in liver malfunctions. Choleodoron is regarded as being more specific in its action and is mostly employed in the treatment of the liver in conditions, such as some gall-bladder disorders, in which its biliary functions are involved. The length of the time over which Choleodoron is taken by the patient is far longer than that which is associated with a course of many of the drugs used in orthodox medicine, such as, for example, penicillin or one of the sulphonamides. Thus the anthroposophical physician Dr Victor Bott, who has stated that he has treated over five hundred patients suffering from gall stones with Choleodoron, in every case avoiding surgical intervention, has advised that this remedy should be taken by the patient for at least three years. Nevertheless its effects have been described by Dr Bott as 'remarkably rapid in the florid type of patient' although somewhat slower on the 'melancholic type'. These latter are, of course, men and women of the Earth type, briefly descibed on p. 55 in relation to the cardinal organs.

Tin which, as was said previously, is often administered to patients in the naturally potentized forms of a vegetabilized metal, is sometimes prescribed in combination with a dynamized organ preparation which is directed at the particular area of the liver on which the physician wishes to concentrate his therapy. It is in a sense a spagyric remedy of the sort associated with Paracelsus and is believed to exert an effect on the liver which is summed up in the alchemical tag *solve et coagula*, 'dissolve and solidify'. That is to say, it is believed to exert a *solve*, that is a softening, effect on the liver when such a softening is desirable, and a *coagula* forming and hardening, influence when that is what the organ requires.

It is worth adding that anthroposophical physicians sometimes employ remedies derived from tin and other medicines which are believed to influence liver functioning in the treatment of conditions in which orthodox practitioners would think it unlikely that the liver was directly or even indirectly involved. Thus, for example, anthroposophical physicians sometimes diagnose depression as resulting from liver malfunctioning. This might be considered as an extremely out-of-date concept by an orthodox psychiatrist, who would, perhaps, think of it as an anachronistic hangover from the Victorian concept of describing someone in a bad temper as 'being liverish' and treating neuroses with tonics and purges.

Anthroposophists, however, are quite unrepentant. Psycho-somatic processes, they insist, operate in two directions: the mind can produce physical disorders and bodily malfunctions can result in psychiatric disturbances. They are satisfied that liver disorders *can* be the causative factor in cases of clinical depression. They also point out that Rudolf Steiner taught that the liver has other functions than carrying out the gross physiological processes which are amenable to laboratory observation and experimentation; disorders in the former cannot, by definition, be diagnosed by physical means, and consequently an orthodox psychiatrist finds no evidence of liver malfunction if he conducts a physical examination of a depressive patient.

Anthroposophical ideas concerning the part played by the liver and other of the body's organs in the genesis of depression and other 'diseases of the soul' are dealt with more fully on p. 156. At this stage it suffices to say that anthroposophical physicians believe that physical factors can play a causative role in some mental disorders.

As is the case with the heart and the liver, the other two cardinal organs, the lung and the kidneys, are often involved in illnesses affecting mature adults.

With the decline of tuberculosis in the Western world those diseases which most commonly affect the lung in adults tend, with the exception of carcinoma, to be long-drawn-out chronic complaints which greatly reduce the quality of life but which are not usually life-threatening until late in life, if at all. Some of these diseases are easily prevented but can only be cured with great difficulty or not at all. Examples of these abound, and some forms of bronchitis and emphysema spring to mind. Smoking and similar abuses of the respiratory system undoubtedly greatly worsen both these conditions, even when they are not entirely responsible for their genesis. Nothing the physician, orthodox or anthroposophical, can prescribe is capable of alleviating these diseases, and perhaps slowing up their advance, unless the patient is willing, like the cardiac patient, to make changes in his or her way of life.

The most obvious of such changes is the abandonment of smoking. This is not found easy by most of us and the general attitude of anthroposophists is that it is found much easier by those people who remove or greatly reduce the stresses and strains which have resulted in a psychological dependence upon tobacco. Some individuals, it is true, can make a considerable effort of will and give up tobacco without changing the patterns of their lives in any other respect. It seems likely, however, that, as the causes which led to nicotine dependence are still intact, they will manifest themselves in other ways – perhaps as a duodenal ulcer, as insomnia or as a dermatosis.

Once the patient has managed to give up smoking there are a number of orthodox and anthroposophical remedies which may be prescribed for the purposes of ensuring that the effects of the damage already done are reduced to manageable proportions. It is interesting to note that at least one homoeopathic physician with leanings towards anthroposophy uses subcutaneous injections of potentized nicotine for this purpose.

Two widespread forms of chronic illness which strictly speaking are not diseases of the lungs but invariably involve the respiratory system are hayfever and asthma. The former is unquestionably an allergy and allergic reactions would seem to be frequently involved in the genesis of asthma. Any allergy is, of course, a bodily reaction to alien substances, typically alien proteins such as are found in pollen. But while we all react to the presence of foreign proteins in our respiratory systems by, for example, producing increased quantities of histamines, most of us have a reaction which is not excessive – our bodies do not manufacture histamines in such quantities that our eyes swell and weep, our nasal passages become blocked and so on. The essence of an allergic reaction is that it is a perfectly normal process which has got out of control and become ludicrously disproportionate to the particular event – such as the inhalation of small quantities of pollen – which has set it in motion.

Anthroposophical physicians discern a similarity between allergic reactions and abnormal emotional responses to stimuli: a bad attack of hayfever, it is said, can be compared with an individual making a violent physical attack upon another human being on the ground that the latter has an unpleasantly noisy way of drinking beer. Anthroposophists believe that emotions, which are always either at the poles of antipathy or sympathy or, more usually, fluctuating between these poles, are essentially astral functions. It is therefore held that any disproportionate emotional reaction probably indicates an astral spasm which results, somewhat paradoxically, from astral weakness rather than strength; it is pointed out that an analogy to this is the strength of the clutch which a baby exerts on any object within its grasp, the grip being so violent precisely because a baby lacks physical strength. The violent reactions of allergy – weeping, sneezing, swelling and so on – are seen as a manifestation on the physical plane of the same astral weaknesses which manifest themselves in the soul as disproportionately violent emotional reactions. What is needed by the hayfever sufferer, say anthroposophical physicians, is a strengthening of the astral forces in their relationship to the mucous membranes of the upper respiratory system.

The most usual remedy prescribed for this purpose is Gencydo, derived from lemon juice and quince pulp in accordance with indications given by Rudolf Steiner almost seventy years ago, which is usually administered both by subcutaneous injection and as a nasal inhalant. A course of injections is commenced well before the pollen count begins to rise – at about the end of March in Central European countries and the higher latitudes of North America, somewhat earlier in England and the southern United States, and at about the end of August in temperate latitudes of the southern hemisphere – and is continued for five or six weeks. At the same time as each injection is given Gencydo liquid is applied to the mucous membranes of the nose. The use of this liquid is continued throughout the summer months by some, although not all, anthroposophical physicians and, in either case, its employment accompanies a second set of injections given in the autumn. This second series of annual injections would seem to be, firstly, intended to strengthen the astral forces of those sufferers whose hayfever originates from grass pollens for the ordeals of the following spring and early summer, and, secondly, to be of particular help to that minority of patients whose nasal allergies are not, strictly speaking, hayfever but a reaction to the fungal spores which abound in the atmosphere during the autumn.

Such courses of treatment are normally continued for at least three years although Dr Bott has reported that one can usually see some improvement in even the first year; he adds that it is usual for the condition to be completely cured by the end of the third year. None the less, some anthroposophical physicians believe it to be advisable to continue with regular courses of Gencydo, even though many years may have passed since any overt symptoms of allergic reaction.

Gencydo is also frequently employed by anthroposophical physicians in the treatment of asthma which sometimes results, so it is said, from an allergic reaction which has 'turned inward', inducing astral spasms. Such spasms are believed to be always the real cause of asthma and can be induced as a result of an overloading of the motor-digestive system as well as of an interiorized allergy.

As well as Gencydo two other remedies were indicated by Steiner as being of particular value in the treatment of the astral disorder which can manifest itself on the physical plane as an asthmatic attack. These are derivatives of the tobacco plant, Nicotiana, usually employed in a 10x dynamization, and the blackthorn, used in the 5x dynamization. All these have, so Steiner asserted, a part to play in getting the astral forces to relax the excessively tight grip upon their too intimate union with the lungs, which is, of course, the cardinal organ which anthroposophists consider to pertain to elemental Earth. In a sense the astral forces in the asthmatic have become too earthy – their proper element is Air, although they are associated with the other three elements. It is for this reason, to strengthen the Air nature, that one of the remedies commonly given by anthroposophical practitioners to asthmatics is subcutaneously injected at a site close to the kidneys, which are, somewhat curiously, the cardinal organs attributed to Air (see p. 48). Nicotiana, the asthma remedy in question, is also used for the treatment of some kidney complaints.

It will be remembered that, as briefly explained on p. 54, Rudolf Steiner and those medical practitioners who accept his teachings believe that the kidneys have a dual function.

Apart from being responsible for the excretory process which is involved in filtering the blood and passing urine into the bladder, they are held to be responsible for 'renal radiation', the impregnation of food substances derived from the digestive tract with human astral forces. The astral body is thought of as being involved in both functions, excretory and 'radiatory', but in different ways. The excretory function of the kidneys has its origin in the direct action of the astral body upon these organs through the nerve-sense system; renal radiation, the astralization process, on the other hand, is held to be a consequence of a less direct action which induces the astral humanization of alien food substances. Disorders of the kidneys are therefore regarded by anthroposophical physicians as being broadly divided into two categories, the first being concerned with the kidneys as organs of excretion, the second with them in their assimilative, astralizing role.

Before describing some of the treatments used by Steiner's medical followers in dealing with kidney complaints which fall into the above categories it is worth saying something about cystitis which, while it is a disease of the bladder (or, rather, a symptom of a bladder disorder) can sometimes, when the cystitis results from an infection, spread upwards from the bladder to the kidney.

The most usual immediate causes of cystitis are an infection of the bladder, commonly by an organism which lives harmlessly in the bowel but can cause trouble when it reaches the urethra and migrates upwards, and an internal bruising of the bladder in which no bacterial invasion is involved. In both cases cystitis is more likely to occur in women than in men: the nature of normal sexual activity is more likely to cause bruising in women than in men, and it is easier for invading bacteria to reach the bladder of women as the female urethra is much shorter in length than its male counterpart.

In dealing with cystitis anthroposophical physicians have available to them, as always, all the drugs used in orthodox medicine and, in addition to these, a large number of homoeopathic and specifically anthroposophic remedies. Homoeopathic remedies which may be prescribed include silver nitrate 20x and dynamized derivatives of cantharides, the 'Spanish fly' of witches' aphrodisiac potions. In the strength in which it has been employed by the manufacturers of aphrodisiacs cantharides is an extremely dangerous drug, its administration resulting in violent irritation of the bladder and urethra, vomiting and sometimes death. In the dynamized forms in which it is employed by anthroposophic physicians, however, it is completely safe and, so it is claimed, an excellent first measure in the treatment of all bladder irritations. Normally the physician would administer dynamized cantharides by injection, but Weleda manufacture a potentized cantharides derivative in pill form which is sold without prescription in many pharmacies and chemists shops. Some women have found that this provides an admirable first-aid home remedy for cystitis; nevertheless, it is always advisable to take medical advice when suffering from this distressing and often painful condition.

Cantharides is an ingredient in a specifically anthroposophical remedy for cystitis manufactured by the Swiss pharmaceutical company WALA. This, Cantharis comp. Wala, is available in two forms, one intended for oral administration, the other for injection. Another ingredient of this WALA compound is equisetum 3x or 4x, the former being included in the formulation designed to be taken by mouth, the latter in the preparation intended for subcutaneous injection. Equisetum, the common horsetail, is the basis of a number of remedies used by anthroposophical physicians in a variety of kidney complaints including some of those characterized by salt retention and an absence or insufficiency of urine production. Many, but not all, of these diseases are considered by anthroposophical physicians to have their real origin, whatever may be their immediate cause, in a failure of the astral body properly to act on the kidneys through the nerve-sense system.

The horsetail derivatives used in the treatment of these conditions are usually prescribed in fairly low dynamizations in the 6x–15x range. In addition hot compresses are applied to the skin in the region of the kidneys – this seems to provide symptomatic relief and, if Rudolf Steiner was right in attributing the warmth, or Fire, element to the Ego, may also bring forces associated with the Ego into action on the astral body at the level of kidney functioning. Subcutaneous injections of dynamized carbon in combination with an anthroposophical organ preparation are sometimes also given to the patient; these are usually given in the pit of the stomach, that is, in the area between the breast bone and the navel. The carbon component of such an injection might well be derived from the partial combustion of horsetail; this would supposedly result in the 'airy' action of the potentized carbon being specifically directed towards the kidneys.

The conditions to which the above treatments are applied are believed, as was said above, to result from an inadequate action of the astral body, via the nerve-sense system, upon the kidneys. Precisely the opposite malfunction, an excessively strong astral impulse through the nerve-sense system resulting in overactivity of the kidneys, can, said Rudolf Steiner, result in a situation favourable to the development of chronic nephritis. Steiner indicated that in such cases, marked by the kidneys' excessive excretions, the physician should endeavour to strengthen the assimilative functions. There is believed to be a subtle planetary relationship between the kidneys and metallic copper and its compounds,[2] and anthroposophical physicians frequently prescribe medicines derived from copper to patients whose excretory kidney functioning seems too pronounced. These include vegetabilized metals, such as copper through camomile and copper through melissa, copper ointments, and ordinary metallic copper in the fourth decimal potency. The inevitable horsetail is also employed, sometimes in combination with copper, more commonly with sulphur, in dynamizations ranging from 3x to 10x.

The assimilative functions referred to above pertain to the renal radiation aspect of kidney functioning, the very existence of which is not accepted by orthodox practitioners, who do not agree with the anthroposophical conception of the human astralization of alien food substances, notably the compounds of proteins. Nevertheless, anthroposophical physicians aver that weak kidney radiation, normally accompanied by an incomplete breakdown of proteins in the digestive system, can manifest itself as a number of symptoms seemingly unrelated to the kidneys, such as arterial hypotension, low blood pressure – shortness of breath, and even the production of large quantities of methane and other gases in the intestines. More directly associated with the kidneys, and also associated with renal radiation by anthroposophical physicians, are some varieties of albuminuria, the presence of significant amounts of water-soluble proteins in the urine. Conversely, it is averred that too strong a kidney radiation can be the real cause of symptoms varying from high blood pressure to cramps and meteorism – a somewhat archaic medical term for the extreme gaseous distension of the upper reaches of the digestive system.

Rudolf Steiner, who made a considerable number of suggestions regarding the treatment of both excessive and insufficient kidney radiation, indicated that the root of the camomile plant would provide a source of remedies for the former condition. As, he said, the root has a certain relationship with the Paracelsian salt principle, it also relates to the nerve-sense system, while the fact that it is strongly alkaline gives it an affinity to the 'watery' etheric body. It is thus considered to be a suitable basis for the preparation of dynamized medicaments designed to harmonize astral and etheric functions and is frequently employed by anthroposophical physicians for such purposes.

Remedies employed in anthroposophical therapy for the opposite condition, weak renal radiation and consequent inadequate astralization of food substances, include dynamized preparations of iron and arsenic – it will be remembered that Steiner averred that 'to give arsenic is to astralize' – both of which are on occasion combined with organ preparations.

Most anthroposophists believe that many of both the major and minor defects of the cardinal organs which have been described above will not occur, or their occurrence will be of a much lesser degree of severity, in adults who follow a natural way of life. As has been pointed out earlier, anthroposophists understand the word 'natural' in a much wider sense than that in which it is commonly employed by, say, wholefood enthusiasts or even devotees of such systems of alternative medicine as naturopathy. It is possible, they say, to be living a thoroughly healthy life in the sense that one avoids junk foods, eats organically grown vegetables, does not smoke, drink or indulge in drugs, takes the optimum amount of physical exercise, and so on, and still be following an unnatural lifestyle which can eventually result in acute or chronic illness. For unless those aspects of existence which are concerned with poetry, music, the arts and the things of the spirit – the life of the soul – are developed in the individual human being, he or she will be living an unnatural life which may eventually manifest itself on the physical plane. If the soul is denied the food appropriate to it, it will grow stunted and deformed as surely as physical starvation will be productive of similar bodily defects. The aim of anthroposophists is, therefore, to provide themselves with a diet which adequately feeds body, soul and spirit.

The first of these goals, ensuring that the body receives nourishment which is both enjoyable to eat, not merely palatable, and adequate for its needs, is in some ways more easily attainable than was the case twenty or thirty years ago. It remains true that biodynamically grown food, or meat from livestock raised in accordance with biodynamic principles, is obtainable only at considerable trouble and expense save by those who live near a farmer or market gardener who conducts his business in accordance with the agricultural and horticultural principles enunciated by Steiner. On the other hand, however, shops selling wholefoods and organically grown cereals, vegetables and fruit – these are considered by most anthroposophists to be the next best to biodynamic products – have proliferated in recent years and are at the present day to be found in most small towns and even in some villages.

Those of us who cannot, for one reason or another, habitually buy the organically grown foods available in such shops can, at least, find a surprisingly large range of wholefoods in many large supermarkets. Thus, for example, 100 per cent stoneground wholemeal loaves, at one time only to be found in a few small bakers' shops, are now supplied by most of the multibranch supermarket chains. There is no doubt that this has resulted from the current vogue for a high-fibre diet, which there are strong reasons to believe may result in a lowered risk of not only bowel diseases, from piles to cancer, but of arteriosclerosis. In this connection it is interesting to note that at a time when orthodox medical practitioners and eminent nutritionists were alike assuring the general public that white bread, provided it was reinforced with iron, calcium compounds and synthetic vitamins, was a thoroughly desirable article of diet, many anthroposophists were arguing to the contrary. Not only, they said, were the bran and wheatgerm which were removed in the milling of white flour of nutritional importance, but these were living substances which could not be fully replaced by chemical and synthetic substances. White bread, they claimed, was subtly devitalized by the processes involved in the manufacture of the flour from which it was made and, consequently, was to be considered as an unsatisfactory substitute for wholemeal bread in a very similar way as manufactured baby foods are considered unsatisfactory substitutes for mothers' milk.[3]

The man or woman who eats biodynamically grown food, avoids stress and provides him or herself with the appropriate mental and spiritual nourishment is regarded as much less likely to suffer from either major or minor illness than the generality of his or her fellows. Nevertheless, none of us can completely cut ourselves off from the stresses and strains of the society in which we live, and those who follow what the medical devotees of Rudolf Steiner believe to be a natural and healthy way of life are not totally immune to the headaches, sleeplessness, colds and other inconveniences which affect the rest of humanity.

Except where such minor complaints are of exceptional frequency or severity, in which case a qualified practitioner is consulted, it is considered by anthroposophical physicians that they can be very adequately dealt with by the home remedies manufactured and sold by anthroposophical pharmaceutical companies – at the time of writing there are in the world no less than twenty-eight of these. The products of these companies include not only specifically anthroposophical medicines but a full range of homoeopathic medicines prepared in accordance with anthroposophical pharmaceutical principles – that is to say, they are not only dynamized by succussion and trituration but their manufacture is conducted in a particular way designed to take account of cosmic influences exerted by the earth, the sun, the moon and the planets.

There are far too many of even specifically anthroposophical home remedies to provide anything like a full listing of them. Those which seem to have the most general appeal and enjoy a large sale in healthfood stores and pharmacies include a copper ointment intended for the relief of muscular pain, a birch elixir, used by many as a spring and autumn tonic as well as for alleviating the pains of muscular rheumatism, ointments and lotions derived from the resin of larch trees and used for the relief of 'tired eyes', and Combudoron, a mixture of tinctures of arnica and nettles which is employed as a dressing for minor burns and scalds. In addition to anthroposophical family remedies and ethical medicines, that is, those not advertised to the general public and supplied only on medical prescriptions, most of the twenty-eight companies mentioned in the preceding paragraph[4] manufacture and/or distribute natural toilet preparations, such as skin lotions and shampoos, compounded in accordance with the pharmaceutical principles formulated by Rudolf Steiner.

While it is believed by anthroposophists that an adherence to a natural lifestyle is productive of a longer and qualitatively better lifespan, nothing, of course, can prevent the inevitable physical wear and tear of life and the onset of old age. The attitude of anthroposophical physicians to the problems associated with ageing is, however, somewhat different to that of their more orthodox colleagues. This is because, in accordance with the teachings of Rudolf Steiner, they do not accept that men and women are no more than uniquely intelligent animals, close relatives of chimpanzees and other primates who have been able, because of the physical development of their brains, to develop languages and exert some control over their environment. They believe that there are qualitative as well as quantitative differences between humanity and even the most intelligent of animals. It might be possible for a behavioural psychologist to devise a language, not necessarily a vocalized one, which would enable, say, chimpanzees to communicate with one another

and with human beings; it might be possible to teach those
same chimpanzees to perform complex tasks; it might one
day be possible to carry out sophisticated surgical procedures
which would give chimpanzees the outward appearance of
humanity: but the qualitative difference between human
beings and chimpanzees would remain unaltered – animals
have no Ego, no central spiritual core which is the ground
of their being.

It is for this reason that, as was mentioned in an earlier
chapter, anthroposophists do not believe that men and
women resemble animals in reaching some sort of developmental peak at the time they reach sexual maturity; on the
contrary, they can, whatever their physical condition,
continue to progress through maturity and old age. There is
no real need, it is said, for those who have reached an age
at which there is inevitably some physical deterioration to
feel that it is now 'downhill all the way', that a stiffness of
the joints must be always accompanied by a stiffness of the
mind, let alone of the spirit.

While the mind can, and should, remain supple and active
throughout old age this is not true of the brain, the physical
focus of consciousness, and the material body of which it
forms a part. There is, so it is believed, a certain 'hardening'
process which is at work in every human being from birth
and, as life goes on, this hardening process becomes dominant over the 'softening' process of growth and cell proliferation which is so noticeable in childhood and adolescence.
This sclerotic tendency most obviously manifests itself in the
appearance of the skin. A young child's skin has a supple
elasticity and an appearance indicative of the abounding
etheric growth forces which are situated just beneath its
surface; the skin of a mature adult has a more mineralized
appearance, suggestive of a hardening process, of a lessening
of the energies responsible for renewal and regeneration, and
the skin of the very old, however carefully looked after, has
a certain leathery scaliness – almost a deadness – which has
come about as a result of natural sclerotic changes.

While the skin provides the most easily discerned of the
symptoms of a sclerosis of ageing, the hardening is of a
general nature and, although it may be slowed down or

temporarily arrested, is irreversible. The jelly-like substance in the eyeball, involved in focusing, becomes harder and more crystalline, resulting in an inability to focus on nearby objects without the aid of spectacles, the joints become stiff, the arteries become sclerosed, sometimes affecting the supply of blood to the brain and resulting in the latter becoming a less efficient medium of communication between mind and body, and so on. Extracts derived from birch leaves and preparations of dynamized lead are the principal weapons of anthroposophical physicians in the struggle to slow down and, for a time, arrest the hardening processes which are regarded as being inseparable from old age and only pathological in nature if they are excessive.

Lead, like other heavy metals, is extremely poisonous (see p. 76) in even quite small doses, but it will be remembered that in the forms in which it is administered by anthroposophical practitioners – usually as dynamized lead acetate, 'sugar of lead', in potencies between 12x and 30x – it is quite harmless, few or none of the original molecules of the lead salt remaining and the remedy being the 'lead process' rather than the metal itself. Dynamized lead is normally administered to the patient in an elixir derived from young birch leaves. This extract may also be prescribed on its own; so may be a tisane derived by infusion from the same leaves either fresh or dried.

As was said earlier, many devotees of anthroposophical medicine consider it advisable to take throughout their entire lives a course of birch-leaf elixir in both the spring and the autumn. This is in total accordance with the anthroposophical attitude towards the hardening, sclerotic diseases of old age. Sclerosis is regarded as a process which normally becomes pathologically apparent only in later life, but it is one which can have its beginnings in early childhood, in adolescence or in the early stages of maturity. It is, in fact, never too early in life to take steps which should prevent pathological manifestations of sclerosis in old age. A too early development of the intellectual powers or sex life of the individual, the excessive bombardment of the soul with sense impressions, the ingestion of devitalized foods and the neglect of the spiritual side of life can, either separately or in combination, result in an early onset of sclerotic diseases of both body and soul.

The anthroposophical approach is, as always, holistic. The quality of the last years of our lives must inevitably be at least partially determined by the nature of the lives which, on the basis of our own free will, we have chosen for ourselves.

PART THREE

Rudolf Steiner, Depth Psychology and the Future of Anthroposophical Medicine

6

Sick Minds, Healthy Minds

A surprisingly large number of otherwise well-informed people do not seem to have even heard of anthroposophy, let alone to have some idea of its teachings concerning mankind and its relationships with other life forms and the mineral kingdom. The name of Rudolf Steiner seems rather better known than that of the movement which he initiated. He is usually vaguely presumed to have been some sort of educational and artistic theorist, a man whose ideas inspired the abstract paintings of Kandinsky,[1] numerous schools such as Michael Hall, and the 'villages' of the international Camphill Movement, known for its communities in which the mentally handicapped villagers live and work with non-handicapped co-workers.

The Camphill Movement, with which many anthroposophical physicians are closely associated, now has about sixty communities worldwide, of which roughly half are in the British Isles. Its origins, curiously enough, are to be found in certain differences which first arose in the General Anthroposophical Society in the period of ten years or so following Rudolf Steiner's death and which were not finally resolved until the middle of the 1960s. These differences resulted in the majority of the anthroposophists of both Holland and Great Britain forming national anthroposophical societies which were quite independent of the worldwide General Anthroposophical Society, which had, and still has, its headquarters at the Goetheanum in Switzerland. The English and Dutch dissidents were joined by a small number of German-speaking anthroposophists. Amongst these latter was Dr

Walter Konig, who founded a small home for the mentally handicapped children at Camphill on the east coast of Scotland shortly before the outbreak of the Second World War.

After the death of any leader – particularly one concerned, like Rudolf Steiner, with spiritual teachings – one or other of two contrasting processes is usually apparent amongst those who have been the dead man's pupils. Either there is a fairly rapid reaction against the previously overwhelming influence of the leader and major revisions are made to the organizational structure of the group he or she has founded and/or led, to the nature of what the group teaches, and to the way those teachings are expressed. Or, perhaps more commonly, there is a period of retrenchment and stabilization, sometimes extending over many years, during which a praiseworthy loyalty to the former leader's teachings sometimes results in a rather mechanical codification of them. This codification can be carried to the point where an adherence to every jot and tittle of the letter of the teachings leads to ossification – a situation in which there is a suspicious rejection of any concept, any way of working, which was not specifically taught in the lifetime of the dead founder. This rejection even extends to ideas and working methods which most unprejudiced observers would consider to be in every way compatible with the original teachings.[2]

It was the latter process which was clearly at work in the worldwide General Anthroposophical Society during the quarter of a century or so following Steiner's death. Fortunately its founder had endowed anthroposophy with some of his own abounding life – I use the last word in its widest sense – so, far from the process of ossification reaching a stage at which the General Anthroposophical Society went into a terminal decline, all that was apparent was a certain rigidity, a tendency to face inwards, rather than to look firmly outwards with the object of extending to new fields the application of Steiner's principles.

This rigidity was much less marked amongst the dissidents, amongst whom, as previously mentioned, Dr Konig, founder of the Camphill Movement, was numbered. He was thus able to enrich his personal concept of anthroposophy with ideas drawn from other sources. These ideas were very largely concerned with the nature of organic human communities in which the whole is greater than the sum of the parts, and those whose lives and writings particularly influenced Dr Konig included John Amos Comenius, Robert Owen and, most important of all, Count Zinzendorf. The first and last of these had been leading figures in the Moravian Church – Dr Konig's wife came from a Moravian family – or *Unitas fratrum*, which had originated in the fifteenth century and combined an ethical approach which clearly derived from the Sermon on the Mount with a theology virtually identical with that of the English Lollards.

Comenius, who died in 1670, had been the last bishop of the old, much persecuted Moravian Church, which had led an underground existence inside Bohemia, and an educational reformer whose ideas about pedagogic methods in some ways anticipated those associated with anthroposophical education. He believed that children should not only be taught classical languages and other academic subjects but singing, arts and crafts. Furthermore he believed that the school should be a world in miniature, with each individual pupil being considered a component part of a living organism, not as a puppet to be drilled in accordance with the schoolmaster's will. Comenius was the last representative of old Moravianism – although one profoundly influenced by the mystical theology of Jacob Boehme – while Count Zinzendorf was the founder of a renewed Moravian Church which came into existence in 1727 on the count's estate in Saxony. It is unlikely that Zinzendorf's particular brand of pietism greatly interested Dr Konig, but he was greatly impressed by the count's advocacy of a community of committed sisters and brothers in Christ sharing in every task, including manual labour. Count Zinzendorf was something of an enthusiast for the latter, particularly where others were concerned, and on one occasion when visited by John Wesley induced the future Patriarch of Methodism to cease holding forth on the errors of Thomas Broughton and instead to dig his, Count Zinzendorf's, garden.

Robert Owen, the early nineteenth-century pioneer of trade unionism and the cooperative movement and the third major non-anthroposophical influence on Dr Konig, was a universalist who believed that all men and women were destined for eventual salvation. It is thus certain that he would not have approved of the theology of either Comenius or Zinzendorf. What he had in common with these two Moravians was a belief that men and women are both happiest and most efficient when living in communities.

At Camphill Dr Konig applied his 'communitarian anthroposophy' even more successfully than Zinzendorf had applied his communitarian Moravianism in Saxony or Robert Owen his communitarian capitalism in the cotton mills of New Lanark. Those who worked with him, not all of them committed anthroposophists, were inspired by his approach to the mentally handicapped. This was based on love and a belief that such individuals were capable of a much greater development than was usually considered possible if they were regarded as being the brothers and sisters of the 'normals' with whom they lived and not as 'clients' of an efficient but largely impersonal system. Whatever the truth or falsehood of Dr Konig's conception of Rudolf Steiner's spiritual science, there is no doubt that the techniques he employed at Camphill – techniques derived from a personal synthesis of anthroposophy and communitarian theory – were effective. Handicapped human beings, who had sometimes been looked upon as little more than sentient vegetables, demonstrated that they were personalities in their own right, capable of making a genuinely valuable contribution to the life of the community of which they were part.

Dr Konig, like other anthroposophists, believed in reincarnation and karma, a spiritual profit-and-loss account carried forward from one life to another. As a consequence of this he held that, whatever the immediate, predisposing causes of congenital mental or physical handicaps (for example, a chromosomal deficiency in individuals suffering from Down's syndrome, formerly known as mongolism), the final causes had to be largely sought in the events of a previous life or lives. This belief, although a very ancient one, was directly derived from Rudolf Steiner who, as was mentioned in chapter 2, attributed Hanz von Hartmann's crippled knee to the karmic consequences of events which had taken place at the time of the Crusades. Similarly, Steiner believed the

insanity of the philosopher Friedrich Nietzsche's later years
to have been a consequence of a previous incarnation as a
Franciscan friar who had practised such austerities that he
had been in continual physical pain. The karmic memory of
this led the Ego of Nietzsche to try continually to part
company with the physical/etheric complex but, being held
within its grip by the abounding vitality of that complex, the
eventual result was insanity.[3] Some critics of Rudolf Steiner
have pointed out that Nietzsche's insanity was almost
certainly a symptom of GPI, tertiary syphilis of the brain.
This, in fact, does not invalidate Steiner's claim for, whatever
the immediate cause of Nietzsche's insanity, the final cause,
which resulted in GPI rather than, say, an aortic aneurism,
could still have been some karmic factor.

It must not be thought that anthroposophical physicians
advocate a crudely mechanical interpretation of karma in
which congenital defects are automatically assumed to be
punishments for sins in a past life in a way similar to that
in which some Fundamentalist Christians think of gout as
God's punishment for gluttony or venereal diseases as God's
punishment for lechery. What is believed, first, is that all of
us must at some stage face the consequences of our actions
in this and previous lives and, secondly, that an incarnating
Ego of its own free will sometimes chooses a defective vehicle
for a particular physical incarnation in order to redeem some
previous failure or to prepare and strengthen itself for tasks
to be undertaken in future lives.

Whether reincarnation is a myth or a reality and whether
Down's syndrome is or is not a consequence of karmic
factors must always be matters of opinion. What is unques-
tionable is that in the many urban and rural communities
which have derived from Dr Konig's original foundation
at Camphill the existence of such beliefs has enormously
strengthened the bonds which unite the handicapped villagers
and the anthroposophical co-workers with whom they share
their lives. For many of the latter hold that in their relationships with the villagers they are, in a sense, renewing old
friendships – re-establishing karmic ties from a previous life
or lives.

Therapy is not regarded as something to be *administered*

to Camphill villagers, be they children or adults – indeed, to regard villagers as being in any sense patients would be the very obverse of the Camphill Movement – but as something that is part of work, play and every other aspect of community life. Thus work in a greenhouse pricking out seedlings is therapeutic, so is candle making, so is the play between an extrovert victim of Down's syndrome and a withdrawn, even autistic child, and so on.

It must be emphasized that while the Camphill Movement came into existence as the result of the work of Dr Konig and other men and women who had been deeply influenced by the teachings of Rudolf Steiner, it is in no sense a subsidiary of the Anthroposophical Society; nor, indeed, are there any formal organizational links between the Camphill Movement and any anthroposophical body. Nevertheless, most of the permanent co-workers in Camphill communities accept the validity of Steiner's spiritual science and many of them are, in their personal capacities, member of the Anthroposophical Society.[4] Thus the Camphill Movement, while independent of anthroposophy, provides an excellent example of the therapeutic application of the principles which underlie anthroposophical medicine.

Severe congenital mental handicap is an affliction suffered by only a small minority of human beings, and anthroposophical attitudes towards its origins and the ways in which its effects can be mitigated is of only theoretical interest to most of us. Nevertheless, it illustrates the fact that the holistic approach associated with the practice of anthroposophical medicine extends not only to the events and circumstances of our present existence but to those of previous lives.

Of more immediate interest to most of us are anthroposophical insights into insomnia and other disturbed patterns of sleep, for these are now very widespread in the Western world and a majority of people have experienced them at some time or another. In this connection it is interesting to note that in a lecture given to medical practitioners and students in 1920 Rudolf Steiner specifically predicted that there would be an 'epidemic of insomnia' in the second half of the twentieth century.

As was stated in an earlier chapter, Rudolf Steiner taught

that sleep was a withdrawal of the Ego and the astral body from the physical/etheric complex – or, rather, of the Ego and that part of the astral body connected with the nerve-sense system. Such a withdrawal can be partial. In full withdrawal there is complete unconsciousness, dreamless sleep; in semi-withdrawal there is dreaming sleep of the type recent psychological research associates with REM (rapid eye movements); in cases of only slight withdrawal daydreams and states of being 'half asleep all through the day' are characteristic.

These latter conditions are, so anthroposophical physicians affirm, very frequently associated with insomnia – the sufferer is rarely fully asleep at night and equally rarely fully awake during the day. In anthroposophical terminology a person afflicted in this way would be considered to have an Ego/upper astral complex which had difficulty in both fully withdrawing from the physical and etheric vehicles and in properly uniting with them. It is considered that there are many possible causes of such a condition but the most common are, first, a disturbance of the organism's rhythms resulting from the artificial nature of present-day urban life and, secondly, a failure to recognize the existence of a spiritual dimension to life and consequently a fear of entering the spiritual world.

The first of these causes, the rhythms of the individual life becoming out of phase with those of nature, has only become a serious problem since widespread industrialization and the increase in the standard of living which has resulted from it. Thus even forty or fifty years ago all save the very rich were far more directly conscious of the rhythmic pattern of the seasons than is the case at the present day. With neither central heating nor air conditioning they directly experienced the coldness of winter and the heat of summer for every hour of the day. Without frozen foods even the most urbanized were vaguely aware of the seasonal cycle of farming and husbandry. For a few months fresh peas were generally available, for a few weeks soft fruit and new potatoes, and so on. This is no longer the case and we have become alienated from the annual solar cycle which runs from one spring equinox to the next; unlike our ancestors, we no longer differentiate between the foods we eat in spring and autumn, the hours we sleep at the two solar solstices, and the pace and length of the working day in summer and winter.

Just as the nature of modern urban life has cut us off from direct links with the great annual solar cycle of germination, growth, harvest and winter rest, so it has disrupted the patterns by which daily life moved in harmony with the twenty-four-hour solar cycle. Our homes no longer show such variations of temperature between day and night, we have no need to slow down the pace of our activity as dusk falls, and many of us turn night into day. But our Circadian rhythms do not easily adjust to such human rearrangements of solar time and, for example, our bodies often continue to make those temperature adjustments appropriate to sleep when we are still active, or those appropriate to activity when we are trying to sleep. The inevitable result is a combination of insomnia and, at other times, sleepiness.

According to anthroposophical physicians, the second major cause of the epidemic of sleeplessness so accurately foretold by Steiner is a fear of the world of the spirit which arises from the application of a mechanistic, reductionist approach to the rich phenomena of life. Those who adopt this point of view, seeing other human beings as a complex combination of cells in which brains excrete thought as livers excrete bile, are caught in a logical trap. For while it is easy enough to regard everyone else in this way it is virtually impossible genuinely to apply this reductionist approach to oneself; for on each occasion one uses the word 'I' in such phrases as 'I think' or 'I feel' one is affirming one's existence as an entity which is more than an aggregation of complex organic molecules. In the words of the anthroposophical physician Friedrich Husemann: 'The man who sees his neighbour as only an aggregate of atoms cannot have the same conception of his own real self. He thus necessarily reaches a position at which there is a fundamental contradiction in his thought.'

A man or woman who endeavours to mask this fundamental inner contradiction, to continue to feel that a mechanistic interpretation of life is a tenable position, can only do so not only by verbally denying the things of the spirit but also by *atempting to avoid every situation which would bring home the reality of the spirit world to him or her*. There is, in fact, a fear of sleep, of detaching the Ego and the astral body from the physical/etheric complex, which arises from the intellectual position which has been adopted. In the first place, the insomniac fears sleep because he or she feels that it is no more than unconsciousness, a 'little death', an entering into emptiness; in the second place, he or she fears it because to sleep is, in effect, to recognize the existence of the world of the spirit and thus to reinforce the fundamental contradiction between reductionism and the act of spiritual affirmation involved in using the word 'I'.

The anthroposophical physician Victor Bott claimed that in those of his patients suffering from sleep disturbances arising from this cause there was often an unavowed longing for spiritual nourishment. So strong was this, he said, that as little as five minutes a day devoted to the practice of some of the simple meditative exercises devised by Rudolf Steiner restored a normal sleep pattern in many of these patients.

Anthroposophical physicians do not believe that psychological states are the causative factor in all cases of insomnia. Rather surprisingly, they attach considerably more importance to physical conditions than do many orthodox practitioners. Thus it is considered that organic lesions, too insignificant to be detected by normal functional and laboratory tests, are sometimes the cause of sleep disturbances which orthodox practitioners have diagnosed as resulting from mental stress, anxiety and other psychological causes. In such cases the minor lesion is treated by administering an anthroposophical remedy appropriate to the particular organ which the physician has diagnosed as being possibly involved in the, seemingly exclusively psychological, sleep disturbances.

It is often found by anthroposophical practitioners that insomniacs have over many years become habituated to the use of sleeping tablets of one sort or another, from mild sedatives to powerful barbiturates, and have developed not only a physical but a psychological dependence upon them. The use of such hypnotics is regarded as extremely undesirable save in cases where the patient is suffering pain of such severity that normal healthy sleep is virtually impossible; as one anthroposophist has said, sedatives no more cure insomnia than aspirins and other analgesics cure a rotten tooth. It is usually found that in many cases of such dependence it is possible to wean patients from their reliance upon hypnotics in the surprisingly short period of two or three weeks, particularly if treatment designed to deal with the causes of insomnia is combined with the use of anthroposophical 'first-aid' remedies for sleeplessness. Medicines of this sort include dynamized *coffea tosta* (roasted coffee) usually administered in the sixth, tenth or twelfth decimal potencies, aconite 20x – found particularly effective in some anxiety states – and belladonna 20x.

Excessive eating at a late hour is also considered as a physically causative factor in some cases of sleep disturbance. On the face of it this seems somewhat surprising, as most of us feel rather sleepy after a large meal. Anthroposophical physicians point out, however, that the sleep which follows overeating is usually a light sleep, frequently disturbed by dreams and nightmares, not the deep sleep which is looked upon as resulting from a proper separa on of the Ego and that part of the body associated with the nerve-sense system from the physical/etheric complex. What has happened when this sort of poor sleep follows on a large meal is, say anthroposophists, that astral forces which properly pertain to the cerebral pole have been called upon to operate at the overloaded metabolic, motor-digestive pole and have thus been unable to accompany the Ego on its separation from the physical and etheric bodies.

Another cause of sleeplessness connected with the digestive processes is very similar to that which, as was explained in chapter 2, anthroposophical physicians believe to be an important factor in triggering migraine – the passage from the digestive system into the organism proper of food substances which have not been fully stripped of non-human etheric forces. In a sense those who suffer from insomnia of this sort, that is, as a result of the Ego and the astral body becoming involved in interior processes which should have been carried out in the digestive system, are victims of a sub-acute migraine of which the symptoms are sleeplessness

rather than pain. In such cases anthroposophical practitioners often find it effective to apply a therapy similar to
that appropriate to migraine itself.

Certain psychologically induced types of sleep disturbances
are treated with the use of physical medicaments, although
very rarely with the powerful psychotropic drugs which are
commonly employed by practitioners of orthodox psychiatric
medicine. Thus insomnia which follows some mental shock,
perhaps, for example, an unexpected bereavement, is quite
frequently treated with dynamized silver. Silver is the remedy
of choice for many supposed disorders of the etheric forces.
It is held that in insomnia resulting from shock a discord has
arisen between the physical and etheric bodies. The silver is
administered, either orally or by subcutaneous injection, in
the 6x dynamization or, in cases where the originating shock
occurred long before the commencement of therapy, in even
higher potencies. It will be remembered that Rudolf Steiner
taught that there is a subtle interconnecting influence
between metals and the sun, the moon and the planets. Such
a connection is believed to exist between silver and the moon,
and it is customary in cases of shock to endeavour to administer potentized silver at a time when the moon is waxing
and the lunar forces are believed to be at their most active.

There are constitutional varieties of insomnia which
anthroposophical physicians classify as being of either a
hysteric or a neurasthenic type. Before considering these one
must first understand in what sense Rudolf Steiner and those
who have studied his teachings on medicine use the words
'hysteria' and 'neurasthenia', both of which are understood
in a much wider sense than in normal psychiatric usage.

Very broadly, for the anthroposophist the neurasthenic is
one in whom the currents of the cephalic pole (which bring
about the breakdown of form) are too strong, while the
hysteric is one in whom they are too weak. Thus hysteria is
a condition in which extra-human forces are active within
the organism because substances which have been ingested
have not been sufficiently broken down, whereas neurasthenia is a condition in which the breaking-down process is
too complete and waste products are, to some degree,
deposited in the organism. To put it another way, hysteria

is characterized by a dominance of the metabolic pole, neurasthenia by a dominance of the cephalic pole.

The insomnia of the hysteric is an insomnia of weakness.
The Ego and the astral body are weak at the cephalic pole
and, precisely because they sense their weakness, they cling
desperately to their hold upon the physical and etheric
vehicles in their nerve-sense aspects. The insomnia of the
neurasthenic, on the other hand, results from excessive
strength of the Ego and the astral forces at the cephalic pole
which results in them experiencing difficulty in relaxing their
grip on the nerve-sense system. This neurasthenic insomnia
is associated, so it is said, with a slowness to become fully
awake in the morning – the cephalic pole awakes easily
enough but the Ego finds difficulty in fully penetrating the
metabolic pole which is associated with the will. As a consequence of this the neurasthenic insomniac becomes conscious
and capable of ordinary thought when he or she rises, but
the lack of will to put thought into action results in him or
her experiencing difficulty in 'getting going' in the morning.

Anthroposophical physicians frequently use dynamized
medicaments to treat both varieties of constitutional
insomnia. Thus a phosphorus salt in an extremely high
potentization, 23x and above, may be prescribed for the
neurasthenic patient to take upon retiring to bed; this is
believed to disperse the forces of the Ego, to drive them
into the spiritual world experienced in deep sleep. The same
medicament in a *low* potentization (5x or 6x) will be taken
by the neurasthenic patient on getting up. It is held that at
these levels phosphorus guides the Ego into the motor-digestive pole and aids a full arousal in which thought is both
ordered and capable of being acted upon. Hysteric insomniacs would find that such medication actually worsened
their condition; for them a tincture of bryophillum, a
member of the stonecrop family in which the etheric forces
are intensely active, is usually the remedy of choice.

It is worthy of note that, as described above, anthroposophical physicians sometimes treat what would usually be
regarded as largely psychological problems with physical
remedies. The same, of course, is true of psychiatric medicine
as it is generally practised at the present day. None the less,

there is a wide gap between the orthodox psychiatrist and the anthroposophical physician. The former does not believe that the psychiatric armoury of hypnotics, antidepressants and other psychotropic drugs can cure his or her patients. All that is asserted is that such drugs can provide symptomatic relief until such time as a spontaneous remission or recovery can remove, wholly or partially, the need for such relief. The psychiatrist also recognizes that most of the drugs used in modern psychiatric medicine are not altogether free of undesirable side effects; in prescribing them the psychiatrist accepts that what is being provided for the patient can never be more than the lesser of two evils.

The anthroposophical physician believes that his or her understanding of the nature of psychiatric disorders is based on a deeper comprehension of the nature of the human organism than is that of orthodox psychiatry or psychotherapy. For him or her the mind is not an illusory epiphenomenon of brain activity; nor are human mental processes the results of changes in brain chemistry; nor are the final causes of psychological illness to be satisfactorily understood on the basis of a materialist, reductionist psychology. The physician who follows the teachings of Rudolf Steiner does not, therefore, administer specifically anthroposophic remedies to those suffering from psychological conditions, such as those associated with insomnia and other disturbances of the mind affecting everyday existence, with the aim of *directly* influencing the physical activities of the central nervous system. It may be, of course, that in certain circumstances the anthroposophical physician would consider it desirable to exert such an influence and in this case he might consider it appropriate to administer one or more of the drugs employed in orthodox psychiatric medicine – for example, lithium to a manic depressive or a barbiturate to a patient suffering from acute insomnia. Nevertheless, it would be considered that all that was being done was to relieve the symptoms of underlying disorders – a barbiturate gives sleep but does not remove the causes of sleeplessness.

Specifically anthroposophical remedies are designed to affect the causative factors in disease, whether of the mind or the body, and in the last analysis all illness is seen as a consequence of disequilibrium and malfunction. If the physico-etheric complex, the astral body and the Ego are all functioning as they should, if the nerve-sense and motor-digestive systems, balanced by the rhythmic system, are acting in harmony, if the processes of inflammation and sclerosis are balanced, then, provided the individual has the physical and spiritual food appropriate to his or her needs, the organism should remain physically and mentally healthy. It must be emphasized that anthroposophists make no sharp distinction between mental and physical illness, one the province of the psychotherapist and the psychiatrist, the other that of the surgeon and the general practitioner. The holistic interpretations of Rudolf Steiner were concerned with the whole human being, body, soul and spirit, and he and those who have come after him have taught that there are physical manifestations of sicknesses of the soul and psychic manifestations of sicknesses of the body. For the anthroposophical physician no illness can be entirely physical or entirely psychological – the Ego, the astral body and the physico-etheric complex continually interact with one another and even a common cold has its emotional (astral) and spiritual aspects.

The anthroposophic remedies employed in the treatment of psychic conditions are, then, prescribed with the intention of restoring the equilibrium of the patient's functioning on all levels, not with exerting a physical effect designed to alleviate or suppress symptoms. For this reason it is quite usual for a medical practitioner who has been influenced by Rudolf Steiner's thought to prescribe for a psychological illness the very same remedies which might be prescribed for a physical complaint. This is illustrated by the nature of the remedies sometimes administered to those suffering from what might be called 'temperamental disequilibrium'.

As was said in an earlier chapter, Rudolf Steiner found the ancient concept of four psychological temperaments, each associated with one of the cardinal organs and one of the elements of Fire, Air, Water and Earth, to be extremely meaningful. It will be remembered that Steiner termed these temperaments choleric (Fire or warmth), sanguine or nervous (Air), phlegmatic (Water) and melancholic (Earth).

In all human beings one or other of the temperaments is believed to be dominant. To the psyche (and to some extent the physical body) of each one of us can reasonably be ascribed an elemental quality which is an outstanding characteristic – we refer to someone as having a fiery temper or an earthy sense of humour, for example. But such a dominance can become so marked that the other elemental qualities, all of which should play a part in the spiritual, emotional and physical life of the individual, are to some extent suppressed. Such a development can become pathological. The fiery person becomes choleric in the colloquial sense of the word, subject to furious rages which can sometimes be of such intensity that violence, mental or physical, results, while the generosity associated with the Fire temperament can become financial and/or emotional recklessness. Similarly the nervous (or sanguine) character can become so Air-dominated that he or she is subject to sudden mood changes of an intensity that disrupts the life of the individual, friends and family. In the same way the phlegmatic, watery, individual can sink into apathy – the fact that we use this watery metaphor is perhaps significant – and the melancholic, the Earth personality, can become both depressed and, in a sense, so heavily laden by the sheer burden of everyday existence that an anxiety state results.

All these temperamental disequilibriums are sometimes treated by the physical administration of anthroposophical remedies. Such remedies will very often be the same as, or similar to, those prescribed for physical disorders of the cardinal organ associated with the particular element which is pathologically overdeveloped in the patient. Take, for example, the choleric, fiery temperament. When this is excessively dominant the individual concerned is violent, this violence sometimes being turned inwards and resulting in suicidal tendencies, reckless and, sometimes, manic behaviour. The Fire qualities of this temperament have, in fact, got out of control – instead of a warming blaze there is a dangerous conflagration. In these circumstances the anthroposophical therapist will remember that the heart is the organ corresponding to Fire and may well prescribe the same, or similar, remedies to those which might be administered to patients suffering from some types of heart disease.

These remedies will almost always include Cardiodoron (see p. 122) and some medicament derived from metallic gold, which is believed, as was said earlier, to have an especial relationship with the heart through certain cosmic influences. In cases in which the choleric excess has resulted in manic behaviour which can be considered as a sort of psychic inflammation, a remedy which is sometimes given for physical inflammation, potentized belladonna, may also be administered. As the Ego, like the heart and the choleric temperament, is considered to partake of the nature of elemental Fire, it may also be judged advisable to transfer some of the activities of the Ego from the cephalic pole to the metabolic pole. To do this the patient who is only tending towards a manic condition may simply be induced to eat a very large meal. In more severe cases vomiting may be induced by one means or another, varying from the administration of tartar emetic to an injection of apomorphine.

Just as the choleric temperament is associated with the heart, so the sanguine, nervous or Air temperament is associated with the kidneys, and some of the medicaments used in the treatment of kidney disorders may be employed in cases involving a pathological 'airyness'. This may well include preparations derived from copper.

A similar situation as far as the administration of physical remedies is concerned prevails in relation to the other two pathological overdevelopments of the temperaments: the depressive, sodden apathy of the Water or phlegmatic individual and the rather different depressive states, often associated with anxiety and phobic states, of the melancholic, the man or woman of Earth. In the former case it is likely that the prescription of the anthroposophical physician will include some of the medicines which are administered to liver patients; in the latter lung medicaments may in some cases be considered appropriate. Hepatodoron (see above) is therefore almost certain to be prescribed for the phlegmatic depressive, as are derivatives of tin. When the depression is of a cyclothymic type, periods of manic exaltation alternating with depressive episodes, a combination of vegetabilized tin with an organ preparation may be administered to the patient during manic phases. Normally the organ preparation is derived from the liver of a young cow, but Dr Victor Bott has made the interesting suggestion that a derivative of a dolphin's liver may be found more effective.[5]

It would seem that in the treatment of the pathological melancholic, in whom the fixity of elemental Earth has become an ossification of the soul, the main aim of anthroposophical therapy is to restore psychic mobility. Hot sulphur baths may be suggested as possibly endowing the patient with some of the qualities associated with the choleric individual and elemental Fire, for warmth is looked upon as mobilizing the Ego. Similarly, mercury, probably in vegetabilized form, can be prescribed, for its quality of fluid mobility is the very antithesis of the earthy rigidity of the melancholic.

It will be noted from the above brief descriptions of the pathological developments of the temperaments that it is asserted that mania can be associated with both the choleric and phlegmatic temperaments. To the outsider this perhaps seems rather odd. Why should two fundamentally contrasting temperamental disorders result in a more or less identical symptom? When I consulted a student of anthroposophical and other holistic therapies on this point it was explained to me that a pathological development of *any* of the four temperaments can result in the cyclothymic disorders which, in their most extreme manifestations, can display themselves as manic depression. While the symptoms of these are very similar to one another, their causes are quite different. In the manic depression of the choleric, for example, it is the fiery mania which is considered to be primary, the succeeding depression being a reaction to this, a consequence of the temporary exhaustion of forces of the Ego by the burning stresses of the manic episode. In the melancholic man or woman, however, the situation is exactly reversed, the depression being primary and the mania a reaction to it.

This seems clear enough, as do the other concepts associated with the anthroposophical version of psychiatric medicine and what might be termed 'physical psychotherapy'. What seems to the non-anthroposophist to be missing from all this is exactly what seems to be missing from Rudolf Steiner's account of the nature of humanity as outlined in chapter 2 – a consideration of the drives, archetypes and so on which are the concern of the depth psychologist, notably the Jungian depth psychologist. I shall endeavour to deal with this seeming omission in my next chapter.

7

Steiner's Cosmogony, the Unconscious and Holistic Therapy

Anthroposophy was once described as 'the occultism of the intellectual'. Such a description is not altogether true, for the breadth of Rudolf Steiner's philosophical vision is such that anthroposophy must properly be looked upon as a conceptual system which subsumes occultism, rather than being a particular variety of it. It remains true, however, that the anthroposophical movement has attracted, and still attracts, men and women of outstanding creative and intellectual ability. One thinks, for example, of the painter Kandinsky, an early pupil of Steiner, of Owen Barfield, the Coleridge scholar, and of Eleanor Merry, who wrote *The Flaming Door*, a much underestimated book. On a more general level it would seem that the average anthroposophist tends to be more widely read, better educated and more aware of contemporary cultural and philosophical trends than do devotees of some other spiritually oriented movements and groupings.

It is not therefore particularly surprising that some anthroposophists have found it disconcerting that there seems to be no room in either the esoteric psychology formulated by Steiner or in the psychiatric therapies associated with anthroposophical medicine for depth psychology generally or, more particularly, the analytical psychology of C. G. Jung and his followers. Some anthroposophists have endeavoured to explain the seeming absence of compatibility between Jung and Steiner with a simplistic tag, 'Jung was concerned with the mind, Steiner with the spirit.' On one very basic level this is a truism – Jung was a psychiatrically qualified physician whose writings were largely concerned with the mind, while Rudolf Steiner was the leader of a religious and philosophical movement and, as such, wrote and talked of 'things of the spirit'. Except on this level, however, the tag is erroneous: for Jung all aspects of psychic activity were in the final analysis spiritual in nature; for Steiner everything, including dense matter, had its origins in the world of spirit and would eventually return to that spiritual state.

This latter idea, that matter is subject to a great cycle of involution/evolution which begins and ends with spirit, is the central concept which underlies every aspect of anthroposophical theory and practice, from education to agriculture and holistic medicine, and is of particular relevance in any consideration of depth psychology in relationship to anthroposophy. Before summarizing this spirit–matter–spirit concept which was presented by Rudolf Steiner in such books as *Occult Science*, and which has been the solid theoretical foundation on which the anthroposophical movement has been built, I think it worthwhile to emphasize two points which must be held in mind when reading this summary.

The first concerns the brief outline, inevitably simplified and schematicized, of Rudolf Steiner's teachings concerning the nature of humanity and the mineral, plant and animal kingdoms over which man has dominion, which was given on pp. 33–60. My concern in that outline was to give the reader the absolute minimum of background information which would enable him or her to appreciate that the practice of anthroposophical medicine is based on an elaborate and internally consistent theoretical structure and is not a mere collection of empirically applied therapies which are employed for no better reason than that Rudolf Steiner suggested that they should be employed. The scheme thus outlined, however, is only a special case, as it were, of the spirit-matter-spirit process which is central to Steiner's cosmology and philosophy.

The second point to be held in mind is that in such books

as *Occult Science* Rudolf Steiner was endeavouring to communicate what must be, to some extent, incommunicable *for those of us who have no access to those modes of perception which he claimed to have.* As a consequence of this he had to use language in an attempt to describe concepts which no words, written or spoken, can altogether satisfactorily express. The way he tried to do this was to employ language in a mode which was neither totally literal nor altogether metaphorical – he used what the old rhetoricians called synedochic speech, in which an aspect of the whole is used to indicate that whole. Thus, when Steiner used the phrase 'Crystal Heaven' in relation to cosmology (thus referring to the Aristotelian concept of successive crystal spheres surrounding the earth, the outermost of which was subject to the direct activities of the Prime Mover, God) he was neither speaking in metaphor nor implying that he accepted the geocentric astronomy of Aristotle and Ptolemy. He was talking synedochically, using a tiny aspect of mankind's understanding of the ultimate reality – Aristotle's concept of the activities of the Prime Mover – to indicate that final reality, from which all else has derived, in its totality.

Before the first manifestation, said Steiner, was the Crystal Heaven, containing a sort of 'process encapsulation' of the events of the evolution which took place before the evolution of our own system began, and 'pure Being' expressing itself as the Spirits of Love, the Spirits of the Harmonies and the Spirits of Will. It seems to be accepted by anthroposophists that these three classes of spirits can be identified with, respectively, the Seraphim, Cherubim and Thrones, which were treated in the *Celestial Hierarchy* of the sixth-century Christian Neo-Platonic philosopher who wrote under the name of Dionysius the Areopagite and who was for long wrongly identified with St Denis of France.

From the primal and timeless state of pure spirit being, the solar system began to come into existence as a 'densification' of spirit, which Steiner called Old Saturn (clearly using that planetary name synedochically) and described as being, at first, 'undifferentiated substance'. At this stage time had not come into existence. Outside Saturn were the three classes of spiritual beings mentioned in the preceding paragraph; within it were the Spirits of Wisdom, Movement and Form. These latter correspond to the spiritual hierarchies of Dominations (Dominions), Virtues (sometimes called Mights) and Powers of Dionysius. Between the two trinities was a sort of differential, insufficient to be regarded as a polarity, which resulted in Old Saturn – that is, all within the zodiac, by which Steiner meant the spiritual gulf separating the highest Dionysian hierarchies from all other aspects of manifestation – beginning to rotate. As a consequence of this rotation, there was initiated a process of separation. Previous to this stage Old Saturn is described by Steiner as being a timeless 'pure warmth of soul'. But separateness manifested itself as a differentiation of the 'warmth of soul' into 'warmth bodies', which Steiner perceived as being the embryonic forms of 'the present physical-mineral body of man, which has evolved out of the old warmth body by [that warmth body] receiving into itself the gaseous liquid and solid substances that only developed at a later stage.'[1] As the warmth bodies became more and more differentiated zodiacal influences resulted in the appearance of the archetypes of physical organs. This curious teaching is of particular relevance to anthroposophical medicine in the context of the supposed relationship, mentioned in chapter 3, between specific human organs and constituent bodies of the solar system. Thus, for example, the Old Saturnian archetype of the heart emerged, said Steiner, under the influence of the zodiacal sign of Leo. The heart, it will be remembered, supposedly has an especial relationship with the sun and, significantly, in traditional astrology the sun is the ruler of Leo.[2]

The Old Saturn stage of development reached its conclusion and there followed a *pralaya* (the word is of Sanskrit origin), which is an interval of rest, more or less identical with what is known in another esoteric tradition as 'a night of the gods'. The warmth bodies, the 'germ of man', said Steiner, entered 'a state of dissolution' which was the same as 'the condition of a plant seed which, resting in the earth, will eventually ripen into a new plant'.

The *pralaya* was succeeded by a solar stage of development, Sun or Old Sun, which began with the germ of man recapitulating the Saturnian evolution and then incarnating itself in 'air bodies'. Just as the prototypes, as it were, of our present day physical-mineral bodies evolved on Old Saturn, so the prototypes of etheric bodies emerged during the Old Sun stage.

Old Sun rotated to a greater degree than Old Saturn and, as a result of complex interactions between it and various spiritual hierarchies, the human prototypes developed the rudiments of the reproductive and other glandular organs. A sort of consciousness developed, similar to that which plants possess in the present day; in old Saturn the warmth bodies had only had a proto-consciousness, which Steiner compared to that of minerals, 'more dim than dreamless sleep'.

Old Sun ended with another *pralaya* which was succeeded by seven epochs of Old Moon, the first two of these recapitulating the Old Saturn and Old Sun evolutions. The prototype human beings now had 'water bodies' and some of them, the most mature, developed astral bodies at this stage. Not all of them were so far advanced and, in Steiner's words,

We find upon Moon forms which are even now [in the period of Old Moon] still at the Saturn stage [i.e. they have prototype physical, but not etheric, bodies] and some also which have reached, but remain, at the stage of the Sun. Two other kingdoms thus emerge besides the properly developed human kingdom. One consists of beings which, having remained at the Saturn stage, have a physical body alone; and this physical body is not yet able, even now on Moon, to become the bearer of an independent [i.e. solar or etheric] body. These beings form the lowest kingdom. . . . A second kingdom is composed of beings who have stopped short at the Sun stage, and are accordingly not ready on Moon to incorporate within themselves independent astral bodies.

Old Moon ended with a period of *pralaya*, similar to that which concluded the Old Saturn and Old Sun stages.

Steiner's scheme is a system of involution as well as one of evolution: it is supposed that spirit 'densifies' and 'condenses' into solidity until a material nadir is reached, at which point the process is reversed, with dense matter 'etherealizing' back towards pure spirit. The nadir is arrived at in the fourth period, that of Earth; we ourselves are held to be living in the fifth cultural epoch of the fifth epoch of this fourth period.

The first two epochs of the Earth period, termed the Polarian and Hyperborean, were devoted to a recapitulation of the Old Saturn and Old Sun evolutions. The Old Moon evolution was similarly recapitulated at the beginning of the third epoch, the Lemurian. During this epoch the densification process continued, although the first Lemurian humanity was still somewhat ethereal, their bodies being 'like plant and flower forms of the most delicate texture'.

In the course of this period there occurred, said Steiner, the event which is semi-allegorically recounted in the story of the Fall of Adam as told in the Book of Genesis. This event was, in fact, the revolt of a spiritual hierarchy collectively referred to as Lucifer. There had been an earlier revolt, that of the hierarchy termed Ahriman, in the preceding period, that of Old Moon. Lucifer always tempts man to pride, egoism in the worst sense, and many Lemurians fell victim to temptation, extending 'the arbitrary power of the fiery spark . . . within them so as to be able to call forth in their environment mighty workings of fire, of a harmful nature. This eventually led to a stupendous Earth catastrophe.' The cataclysm wiped out most of the Lemurians, although certain 'savage tribes' which either still survive or survived into the last century were of Lemurian descent.[3]

The Lemurian epoch was succeeded by that of the Atlanteans, the fourth of the seven epochs of the fourth period and, of course, that immediately preceding our own epoch. As such it came at the exact midpoint of the evolution/involution process and *should* have marked the nadir of descent from spirit into matter. But as a result of the Luciferic rebellion in the Lemurian epoch the process of descent continued past its due time, spirit becoming more and more involved with matter. Things were made even worse by the intervention of the Ahrimanic hierarchy which, it will be remembered, had rebelled against the ordained course of evolution/involution during the Old Moon period.

The Ahrimanic and Luciferic spirits exerted their baleful influences upon the Atlanteans but the effects of these were to some extent mitigated by the strivings of certain initiates, notably those who served the Sun Oracle and had a particular knowledge of the (cosmic) Christ – for Steiner the archetypal 'I', a mighty Spirit Being particularly associated with the Sun. In time, however, even the majority of these initiates were corrupted by the Ahrimanic legions, with the consequence that 'Mighty and ominous powers of nature were ... let loose by the deeds of men, leading eventually to the gradual destruction of the whole territory of Atlantis by catastrophes of air and water'; the last of these catastrophes, the final sinking of Atlantis, took place between ten and twelve thousand years ago.

The end of Atlantis coincided with the beginning of our own epoch, of which we are currently in the fifth of seven cultural epochs, as is shown in the following table:

Fourth 'Earth' period of cosmic evolution and involution

1 Polarian epoch
2 Hyperborean epoch
3 Lemurian epoch
4 Atlantean epoch
5 Post-Atlantean epoch:
   (a) Ancient Indian cultural epoch
   (b) Ancient Persian cultural epoch
   (c) Egypto-Chaldean cultural epoch
   (d) Graeco-Latin cultural epoch
   (e) Our present-day cultural epoch
   (f) Sixth cultural epoch
   (g) Seventh cultural epoch
6 Sixth epoch of Earth period
7 Seventh epoch of Earth period

The 'culture hero' of the first post-Atlantean cultural epoch,[4] the Ancient Indian, was supposedly a refugee from sinking Atlantis and composed the archaic, or archetypal, Vedas, which were the remote ancestors of the Vedas known to oriental scholarship. The Ancient Persians of the second cultural epoch were very deeply involved in the world of matter, exploiting nature for their own, largely selfish, ends. Even more sunk into mere physicality were the men and women of the succeeding Graeco-Latin cultural epoch, which began at the time when Romulus and Remus founded the city of Rome. By this time mankind had sunk so deeply into matter that the process would have become irreversible, a triumph for the Ahrimanic and Luciferic hierarchies, had it not been for the incarnation of Christ, the archetypal 'I'.

The *essential* Christ Being, said Steiner, must not be confused with the identity of the man Jesus of Nazareth or, rather, with the *two* Jesuses of Nazareth. The first of these was the 'Wisdom' or 'Solomonic' Jesus, the Jesus whose origins were described in the Gospel of St Matthew and who was, in fact, a reincarnation of the ancient Iranian prophet Zarathustra. The second was the 'Love' or 'Nathan' Jesus, whose origins were described in the opening chapter of the Gospel of St Luke. At the time of the visit of the boy Jesus to the Temple, as described in St Luke, 2, 41–51, the two Jesuses fused into one, a transformed Jesus into whose body the Christ descended some eighteen years later at the time of the baptism in the Jordan. The transformed body was united with the Christ until the Crucifixion, when the moment of separation was marked by Jesus's cry of 'My God, my God, why hast thou forsaken me?'

Steiner's assertion that Christ was only united with Jesus for the last three years of the latter's ministry has been described by some critics of anthroposophy as a revival of the ancient docetic heresy which was adhered to, in one form or another, by many Gnostic and dualist sects. Strictly speaking this is hardly correct. The docetics believed that Christ had only an illusory, phantom body; Steiner, however, asserted that the body was real although its substance was spiritualized. It would seem that if one wants to find an heretical antecedent for Rudolf Steiner's Christology it should be sought in the Adoptionism of Paul of Samosata, who taught that, at the moment of his immersion in the Jordan by St John the Baptist, Jesus became the *adopted* Son of God.[5]

The Crucifixion, said Steiner, was the turning point in the history of mankind and the cosmos – the 'Cosmos of Wisdom' ascending as the 'Cosmos of Love' and a process of return from matter to spirit being initiated.

The Graeco-Latin cultural epoch finally came to its end shortly after the beginning of the fifteenth century and was succeeded by our own epoch, which is characterized by 'the antagonism between external science and spiritual knowledge' and the emergence of the Rosicrucian mysteries (anthroposophy being considered to be connected with, or even an aspect of, these).

The sixth cultural epoch, towards which our own society is evolving, will witness the Second Coming of Christ, but not in the sense that the phrase would be understood by Christian fundamentalists. What will happen is that more and more human beings will perceive Christ etherically and, as a consequence of this, will be led to accept 'the Knowledge of the Graal', which is the evolutionary goal of that cultural epoch.

In the seventh cultural epoch, wrote Steiner,

the souls who have reached the evolutionary goal of the sixth will go on evolving. For those who have not, even the surrounding world will be too greatly altered [to make up the lost ground]; they will find little opportunity to recover ... and must await a more distant future when the conditions will again be favourable.

The end of the seventh *cultural* epoch and the beginning of the sixth epoch will be marked by cataclysmic events of a violence approaching or even equalling those which resulted in the final destruction of Atlantis.

The involutionary process of respiritualization which began at the Crucifixion will continue throughout the sixth and seventh epochs of the Earth period, by the conclusion of which the earth on which man lives – already transformed by its union with the moon towards the end of the fifth epoch – will have united with the sun and the planets.

After the usual interval of *pralaya* the Jupiter period will succeed. This, of course, will also be divided into seven epochs, the first four of which will recapitulate, one by one, the experiences of the Saturn, Sun, Moon and Earth phases of evolutionary/involutionary manifestation. During the last three epochs the respiritualization continues at all levels, with minerals becoming, as it were, plant-like, and plants becoming animal-like.

After the customary *pralaya* the Venus period begins, the first five of its seven epochs being devoted to the usual recapitulations. During the last two epochs animals are the lowest form of life and above them are three grades of humanity. After *pralaya* comes the final period which Rudolf Steiner termed Vulcan. This was rather an interesting choice of name: Vulcan is the name given to a hypothetical planet which some astronomers supposed to have an orbit inside that of Mercury and the supposed existence of which seemed to account for certain perturbations in the orbit of that planet which were not explicable in terms of Newtonian gravitational theory. These perturbations are now believed to be the consequence of effects predictable on the basis of relativity and today nobody save a handful of astrologers believes in the existence of Vulcan. In view of the nonexistence of the planet Vulcan it seems exquisitely suitable that Rudolf Steiner wrote that any description of the period named after it would be beyond the compass of his book, *Occult Science*.[6]

Such, in outline, is Rudolf Steiner's account of the past, present and future of the solar system and its inhabitants.[7] Of that account in its entirety Maurice Maeterlinck wrote:

Steiner has applied his intuitive methods . . . in order to reconstruct the history of the Atlanteans and to reveal to us what takes place on the sun, the moon and other worlds. He describes the successive transformations of the entities which became men, and he does so with such assurance that we ask ourselves, having followed him with interest through the introductions which reveal an extremely well-balanced, logical and comprehensive mind, if he has suddenly gone mad or we are dealing with a hoaxer or with a genuine seer.

Most readers of Steiner's cosmological and historical writings would be inclined to agree that their author must be categorized under one of Maeterlinck's three classifications. It is perhaps worth remarking, however, that such categories are not necessarily exclusive. Over sixty years ago the writer Gustav Meyrink pointed out that a study of the lives and teachings of many spiritual leaders, past and

present, sometimes reveals an extraordinary element of char-
latanism – even fraud – in even those whose wisdom is
beyond doubt.

Be that as it may, it is worth remembering that while
Rudolf Steiner developed the theories underlying anthroposophical medicine within the framework of his remarkable
cosmology the former is not logically dependent upon the
latter. Thus, for example, it is possible to believe that Steiner
was correct in what he taught concerning the polarity of the
nerve-sense and metabolic-limb systems without having to
believe that he was equally correct in what he said about
Old Saturn. It is also possible to extend this attitude to the
entire theoretical framework of anthroposophical medicine,
although such an approach would not be favoured by
anthroposophical medical practitioners.

Such a pragmatic approach to anthroposophical medicine
is not unknown – I have met a militant communist and
atheist who took Bidor (a remedy compounded on the basis
of indications given by Rudolf Steiner) for her migraine
because she found it to be effective. On the whole, however,
those who regularly use anthroposophical medicines for their
everyday complaints are at least inclined to an acceptance of
the 'irrational' anthroposophical cosmogony which has been
outlined above, while most qualified physicians who practise
holistic medicine on the basis of the indications given by
Steiner are committed to an acceptance of that cosmogony
in its entirety.

It might therefore be considered that the supposedly
irrational elements in this cosmogony are the result of some
fundamental incompatibility between anthroposophy and
Freudian, Jungian and other schools of depth psychology.
However, those acquainted with the history of both
occultism and Freudian and other types of depth psychology
find it difficult to sustain any approach which categorizes
anthroposophy as 'irrational' and depth psychology as
'rational'. There is, in fact, a very curious historic relationship between occultism and those psychological schema
which have been concerned with the Unconscious. Sigmund
Freud himself, while most certainly not an occultist, had
some very strange and enduring connections with the

shadowy world of the occult counter-culture, connections which have very largely been hidden from general view, mainly as a result of deliberate mystifications and reticences on the part of both Freud himself – who seems to have had an almost obsessional concern to show himself as an *original* thinker – and of pious disciples who were anxious that the Master's reputation as a rational thinker should be preserved.

It will be remembered that, as was mentioned in earlier chapters, Eduard von Hartmann published the first edition of his *Philosophy of the Unconscious* in 1868, only twelve years or so after Freud's birth. In view of the still very widely held belief that Freud originated the concept of the existence of the unconscious mind, it is worth emphasizing that, as Lancelot Law Whyte pointed out almost a quarter of a century ago, von Hartmann analysed the supposed contents and functioning of the unconscious mind under twenty-six separate aspects. Von Hartmann, however, was no more the first man to posit the existence of the unconscious mind than was Freud himself.[8] The history of theories concerning the existence of the Unconscious certainly goes back to the seventeenth century and probably much further – one contributor to psychoanalytical publications of the 1930s, a man who had been a friend of Freud since the latter left school, asserted that the Neo-Platonists of the early centuries of the Christian era were well acquainted with the concept. Interestingly enough, the man in question was none other than Friedrich Eckstein, the Viennese admirer of Madame Blavatsky through whom Rudolf Steiner had first been introduced to the writings of A. P. Sinnett and other Theosophical propagandists. It is known that, at the same period of his life at which he was closest to the young Sigmund Freud, an esoteric circle of which Eckstein was the leading light was particularly concerned with the teachings of the Greek philosopher Empedocles. Furthermore, it has been argued, notably by Garfield Tourney, that Freud was heavily indebted to Empedoclean philosophy for the concept – notably present in his later writings – of opposing forces, one desiring life, one death, at work in the Unconscious. It seems at least possible that it was through his friendship with Eckstein that Freud had first come into contact with Empedoclean philosophy. If so, influences deriving from circles directly concerned with esoteric philosophy played a part in the genesis of what are usually considered to be specifically Freudian concepts.

In general, however, Freud displayed an attitude of hostility to the whole gamut of ideas which he generally subsumed under some such description as 'the occult' or 'mysticism'. This hostility was very powerfully expressed in a conversation with C. G. Jung which took place in 1910. 'My dear Jung,' began Freud, 'promise me never to abandon the sexual theory. That is the most essential thing of all. You see, we must make a dogma of it, an unshakeable theory.'

Reasonably enough, Jung asked Freud what the theory was supposed to be a bulwark *against*. Freud replied hesitantly, 'Against the black tide of mud – occultism.' In his autobiography, *Memories, Dreams, Reflections*, Jung expressed his astonishment at this extraordinarily irrational statement by which Freud seemed to be urging him to give his lifelong allegiance to a particular theory concerning the origins of neuroses, not because that theory was necessarily true, but because it was a protection against the 'occult' threat. The wide limits of what Freud included under the blanket term 'mud of occultism' was made clear by Jung: 'What Freud seemed to mean . . . was virtually everything that philosophy and religion, including the rising contemporary science of parapsychology, had learned about the psyche.'

Freud's attitude towards mysticism and occultism was clearly something more than a mere intellectual revulsion: it would seem that he was frightened of it, seeing it as a threat, something against which he and others needed a bulwark. Exaggerated fear of this sort – whether the object of it is homosexuality, occultism or overeating – is usually an indication that the phobic is attracted to that which he or she fears. I do not think that Sigmund Freud was an exception; I believe that he was fearful of the occult because he felt strongly attracted towards it.

There is evidence which, while it does not prove the existence of such an attraction, shows it to have been likely. Such evidence, apart from Freud's connections with Eckstein[9] – who was not only a Theosophist but a student of kabalistic and Neo-Platonic mysticism – includes his early devotion to hypnotism, which at that time was still regarded as semi-occult by most physicians, and his close friendship, from 1887 until 1903, with Wilhelm Fliess, whose numerological speculations would seem to belong to the same class of 'mystical arithmetic' as that with which, as described in chapter 2, some anthroposophical physicians have endeavoured to show a link between, on the one hand, the rhythms of the human cardiac and respiratory systems and, on the other hand, the solar year and the precession of the equinoxes.

Fliess's numerology was based on the belief that besides the (roughly) twenty-eight-day, female, 'lunar' sexual cycle associated with menstruation there was also a twenty-three-day, male, 'solar' sexual cycle. The supposed interaction of these two cycles was used by Fliess, who also believed that all human beings were bisexual and thus subject to the influences of both periodicities, to explain almost every aspect of human life, from episodes of exceptional creativity to the dates of illness and death. There is no doubt whatsoever that for some years Freud was fascinated by this and other of Fliess's theories – for example, the belief that there was a specific *physiological* connection between the nose and the genitals – and attempted to incorporate them into the theoretical structure of psychoanalysis.

Whether or no Fliess developed his theory entirely independently of written sources or other outside influences is neither here nor there – what matters is that similar numerological and cyclical theories had long been associated with the occult tradition. Thus, for example, in 1882 Baron Hellenbach, a man who may have been known to both Freud and Fliess, and was quite certainly known to Friedrich Eckstein, published in Vienna a work which was concerned with numerical rhythmic cycles and displayed an excessive, and probably unwarranted, belief in the significance of the quaternary. Hellenbach's ideas were derived from the numerological theories of the Austrian occultist and medical practitioner, Fritz Liharzik, who was himself intellectually indebted to the writings of the seventeenth-century Jesuit writer Athanasius Kircher, who had been a student of kabalism and the supposed secrets contained in a mysterious 'emblematic Isiac Tablet of Cardinal Bembo', whatever that may have been. It is clear, then, that Freud's friend Wilhelm Fliess was not just a surgeon with odd beliefs about noses and numbers, but a man whose ideas, whatever their source, were related to occult traditions.

Freud's fear of occultism was undoubtedly heightened by his quarrels with associates who had become involved in psychic research, mystical studies and so on. Thus he was annoyed, and probably alarmed, by Wilhelm Stekel's assertions that 'telepathic dreams' – the existence of which Freud believed to be at least possible – disproved one of the most fundamental psychoanalytical concepts, that under a veil of symbolism the content of dreams expressed the dreamer's unconscious desires. Stekel wrote:

The telepathic dream contradicts Freud's theory. It is never a wish fulfilment. So orthodox psychoanalysis does not want to recognize the telepathic dream.
Because of this, Freud and his immediate circle doubt the exist-ence of the telepathic dream. I cannot understand this doubt and am forced to trace it back to a prejudice against all occult questions.

In spite of this supposed prejudice, the pull of the occult was strong enough for Freud to give his approval to a series of telepathic experiments undertaken by his own daughter, Anna, in cooperation with Sandor Ferenczi, the Hungarian analyst who was, until *circa* 1930, one of Freud's closest associates. Ferenczi eventually became so convinced of the reality of telepathy that he underwent, or believed that he underwent, a telepathic analysis.

It was, however, the occult and mystical tendencies of C. G. Jung, the Swiss physician whose *Psychology of the Unconscious* had been so strongly attacked by Rudolf Steiner (see p. 57), which caused Freud the most distress. It was only in 1907 that Jung had become closely associated with Freud and as early as the following year at least one member of the psychoanalytical movement, Karl Abraham, is reported to have warned the Master against the Swiss physician's 'tendency to occultism, astrology and mysticism'. If reports of Jung's own supposed mediumistic powers – almost ten years before first meeting Freud he had been the focus of some poltergeist-like phenomena – had reached Freud, it seems likely that he would have taken Abraham's warning more seriously than he did.

A year later Freud himself experienced curious phenomena in Jung's presence, two mysterious explosive sounds being heard by both men. Jung referred to these as 'catalytic exteriorization phenomena' – in other words, he was saying that some interior psychic force within himself had produced the noises; Freud, more prosaically, blamed the noises on effects involving expansion and contraction produced by the idiosyncrasies of his heating system.

Freud endured Jung's propensity for psychic explosions; what he found himself unable to accept was his associate's growing conviction that the Freudian sexual theory was inadequate. The differences between the two men grew more and more pronounced until finally, in 1913, there was a complete break between them. This break seems to have been the causative factor in Jung undergoing an extraordinary crisis which culminated in poltergeist phenomena, the visit of a crowd of spirits, and the production of a strange but powerful neo-Gnostic text entitled *Seven Sermons to the Dead*.

Jung himself recounted the story of these events in a way which makes it seem uncertain whether he regarded them as more 'exteriorization phenomena' or consequent upon direct contact with objectively existing spiritual beings. In fact, as will be explained later in connection with Rudolf Steiner's criticisms of Jung's attitudes, the latter not only did not regard these categories as mutually exclusive but considered that, in the last analysis, such categorizations are virtually meaningless.

The poltergeist phenomena were certainly objective enough, taking the form of the front door bell pealing of its own accord. Most of us, no doubt, would have suspected the activities of a hoaxer, but Jung felt sure that 'something had to happen', a feeling accentuated by his perception that his home was 'crammed full of spirits' crying out to him in chorus, 'We have come back from Jerusalem where we found not what we sought.'

A variant of the spirits' chorus provided the opening words of *Seven Sermons*, in which Jung, as 'Basilides', expounded what can perhaps best be regarded as a psychological variant of Gnosticism. Like most Gnostic systems, Jung's starts with the 'Pleroma' – the Divine Being and its aeons or emanations – but, untypically, does not provide any real description of this, merely stating that it is 'all', 'nothing' and a thing on the nature of which it is pointless to speculate. In essence, then, the Jungian Pleroma can be identified with both the Pleroma of the ancient Gnostics and the Crystal Heaven which is the starting point of Rudolf Steiner's cosmogony as described earlier. As Jung taught that mankind derives from the Pleroma, that men and women are, in a sense, its emanations, his system again correlates with that of the ancient Gnostics, who conceived men and women as beings in which a certain component of divinity, spirit or light was trapped in an envelope of darkness, physical matter. The scheme of solar evolution described by Steiner and briefly outlined on pp. 161–68, which sees the cosmos as originating in the world of pure spirit, 'densifying' itself into matter and finally returning to pure spirit, is very similar in its essentials.

Where, however, Jung's Gnosticism as outlined in *Seven Sermons* seems to differ radically from both classical Gnosticism and Steiner's teachings concerning human evolution is in its attitude towards the individual's relationship to the totality of the Pleroma. As far as the Gnostics were concerned, the task of the individual was to free the 'seeds of light' from the bondage of matter and reunite them with the Pleroma; as far as Rudolf Steiner was concerned, that same task was to aid the collective return of humanity and, indeed, all manifestation, to the world of primal spirit; but Jung saw the matter quite differently. As far as he was concerned, the essence of humanity was that it was distinct from the Pleroma, and this distinction must be maintained by each and every man and woman – the Jungian principle of 'individuation' is no more than a special case of such distinction maintenance. If the distinction is *not* maintained, said Jung, humanity loses its individuality and falls back, as it were, into the Pleroma.

Seven Sermons, the book in which Jung outlined his neo-Gnosticism, was produced in 1916 by at least 'semi-automatic' writing: Jung wrote it while in a state of partial trance, he did not consciously formulate its structure and argument, and its author was, in a sense, not Jung but some entity *within* him. Whether that entity was an objectively existing discarnate being, as some spiritualists believe, or some aspect of Jung's own mind, or neither, or even both, is of no great relevance; what is important is that *Seven Sermons*, a book which resulted from the use of a technique more usually associated with spiritualist mediumship than with a scholarly application of the scientific method, *is the core text of Jungian depth psychology*. It is possible, one supposes, that by some curious circumstance involving a dissociation of consciousness an authentically scholarly paper or book might be produced by, say, a physicist in trance or semi-trance. But *Seven Sermons* is in no sense a scholarly production; it belongs to the same class of literature as Gnostic apocalypses and, more recent examples of the genre, the 'Holy Books' produced by, or perhaps through, Aleister Crowley. C. G. Jung was well aware of the nature of *Seven Sermons*, as is indicated by the full title and subtitle he gave to the book, *VII Sermones Ad Mortuos: The Seven Sermons to the Dead, Written by Basilides in Alexandria, the City Where the East Touches the West.*

Jung's choice of the pseudonym of 'Basilides *in* Alexandria' was of considerable significance, for the original Basilides, a second-century Gnostic heresiarch, lived and taught in Alexandria although by birth he seems to have been a Syrian. For Basilides the Supreme Being could only be described by negatives – an interesting anticipation of the negative mystical theology of Dionysius the Areopagite which seems to have very possibly influenced Rudolf Steiner – but it was possible, said Basilides, to approach this final source by successively gaining access to the series of 365 gradations of spiritual reality which had emanated from it.

Each letter of the Greek alphabet has a numerical value, and the Basilidean concept of 365 emanations could therefore be expressed by the word 'Abraxas', which is frequently found engraved on Gnostic gems. In *Seven Sermons* Basilides/

Jung used the word 'Abraxas' to represent 'illusory reality'; in the final analysis this usage is compatible with that of the original Basilides, for whom the 365 'heavens' were all, in a sense, illusory, veils which had to be torn aside before the true knowledge of reality could be obtained.

From *Seven Sermons* it is not altogether clear what the dead had 'sought but not found' in Jerusalem. Basilides/Jung undoubtedly believed that they sought much, not all of which it was wise for him to reveal to the world. I suspect that one thing they sought in vain was, in a sense, Christ; for it seems likely that Basilides/Jung shared the heretical Christology of the original Basilides.

The Basilidean Christology was in many ways similar to that of Rudolf Steiner as I have described it on p. 166; Christ was 'Mind', the first and highest emanation of the Supreme God, sent forth to redeem humanity and united with the body of Jesus of Nazareth at the time of his baptism in the Jordan. At the time of the Crucifixion, said Basilides, the Christ spirit, eternal Mind, separated from the body of Jesus and ascended into its own region, leaving the body it had occupied to dissolve into formlessness, for the 'body' which perished on the cross was either an illusory phantom or, according to some accounts of Basilides' teachings, was that of Simon of Cyrene, which had been substituted for that of Jesus.

Some of those who have been deeply influenced by Jung's writings have argued that *Seven Sermons* is little more than an aberration, in no way central to his thought. Such an attitude is understandable but not sustainable. There can be no real doubt that Jung was a Gnostic and that *Seven Sermons*, far from being peripheral to the structure of Jungian depth psychology, is the central core from which all post-1916 Jungian developments have derived. Furthermore there is some reason to believe that Jung had direct associations with one or more neo-Gnostic groupings. In this context a statement made by Jung in relationship to the *Tibetan Book of the Dead* is of great significance. There are no Western equivalents to this book, wrote Jung, 'except for certain secret writings which are inaccessible to the wider public and the ordinary scientist'. The implication seems clear: Jung *knew* of the existence of these writings and therefore must have had access to them. This would not have been the case unless he was an initiate of secret groups and not, as he himself said, either a member of the 'wider public' or an 'ordinary scientist'.

Nevertheless, there are still those who insist that Jung was only concerned with esoteric systems as projections of the mind, that he did not accept their validity external to the psyche, and that he had the greatest contempt for occultists and occultism. Such a viewpoint is often supported by references to Jung's own statements: for example, his assertion that Theosophy is 'indescribably cheap, impoverished and lacking in creative energy', or his protestations that those who criticized him ignored 'the fact that as a doctor and scientist I proceed from facts. . . . Instead they cite me as if I were . . . a Gnostic with pretensions to supernatural knowledge.'

But a contempt for the post-Blavatskyan Theosophical Society is almost a trademark of the intellectual neo-Gnostic – Aleister Crowley, for example, habitually referred to its teachings as 'Toshosophy' – and Jung *did* make pretensions to supernatural knowledge, replying to a question as to whether he believed in the existence of God with the words: 'I don't *believe*, I know.' It is in the light of this statement that one should undoubtedly interpret a statement written by Jung in 1936 concerning the Nazi paganism of the German Faith Movement led by Jacob Hauer. 'There are people in the German Faith Movement', wrote Jung, 'who are intelligent enough to not only *believe* but to *know* that the God of the *Germans* is Wotan and not the Christian God.' In general, however, Jung wrote in such a way as to encourage the belief that his concern was only with interior, psychic realities, not with occult cosmologies as statements of objective truth about the origin and destiny of humanity and the world which it inhabits.

There are, however, certain elements in Jung's writings which make it apparent that he did *not* regard Gnosticism, astrology and other forms of divination, alchemy, the projection of 'spirit bodies' and all the other beliefs subsumed under the term 'occult' as being only psychologically true.

Before considering these elements it is worth pointing out a curious fact which may easily be checked. If one obtains an article or a book written by a practising analyst of any school of depth psychology save the Jungian and goes through it substituting for the words 'therapy' or 'analysis' the phrase 'invocation of the gods by means of ritual magic', and, similarly, substituting the phrase 'spiritual evolution' for the words 'improvement' or 'cure', one ends up with what is clearly a piece of meaningless nonsense. If one follows a precisely similar procedure (save that the word 'individuation' is also replaced by 'spiritual evolution') with almost any lengthy passage from Jung's writings one ends up with a coherent statement which could have been written by almost any twentieth-century practitioner of Western ritual magic. To say this is not to denigrate Jung's writings; it is only to point out that they belong to a tradition which extends backwards in time to classical antiquity, a tradition which is also represented by the writings of Paracelsus and Cornelius Agrippa. I think it worthwhile pointing out that others who derived from that same tradition – 'black' occultists, 'white' magicians and esotericists of all shades of grey – were quick to recognize Jung's true affiliations. Thus as early as 1918 the occultist Aleister Crowley was reading Jung and noting in his diary that as a result of doing so he was in process of developing a new magical technique. Similarly, one of the first Jungian lay analysts in England was a practising ritual magician and chief of an occult temple which was derived from the very same esoteric order which provided Rudolf Steiner with his first English disciples.[11]

The elements in Jung's writings which overtly proclaim his allegiance to occult tradition are those concerned with divination in general and astrology in particular. It is absolutely beyond doubt that C. G. Jung accepted the *objective* truth of astrology: he did not regard it as being simply some 'poetic' symbolic system which could be dispassionately examined to see if it threw light on the nature of unconscious processes, archetypes, and so on, but as a method of accurately delineating character and, to some extent, foretelling the probable course of events. It is, in fact, apparent that Jung was acquainted with astrological writings of considerable obscurity (for example, those produced by 'A. G. Trent', Richard Garnett, once Keeper of Printed Books of the British Museum) and that he had studied the techniques of this occult science as a believer, not as a detached observer.

Why, then, did Rudolf Steiner find the *Psychology of the Unconscious* and the other (early) writings of Jung so offensive? What seems to have misled Steiner, as it has misled some other readers of Jung, was the latter's concept of 'psychic truths'. Jung reiterated again and again that *as a psychologist* he was not concerned with the question of whether gods, demons, angels or a Supreme Being enjoy an 'objective existence'. He wrote: 'The idea of God is simply a necessary psychological function of an irrational nature, which has nothing to do with the question of the actual existence of God.' Rudolf Steiner found the sentiment expressed in this statement to be peculiarly repellent. He wrote:

When you read the complete sentence you run upon the great dilemma of the present day. The psychoanalyst proves to you that man becomes ill and useless without his God, but says that this need has nothing to do with the existence or nonexistence of God. . . . They [psychoanalysts] admit an absolute necessity, but when that necessity is stated as a serious question they consider it one of the stupidest that can be suggested.

The nature of the criticism made by Rudolf Steiner in the above passage seems to make it apparent that he had not realized that Jung was saying that the question 'Does God exist?' is not meaningless in itself, but that it is meaningless *in the context of analytical psychology*, for God, as a 'psychic truth', exists in the mind of every man and woman and therefore *must* exist for the psychologist. God, angels, demons are all psychic truths – which does not mean that they are not 'objectively true' or in some way 'less true' than, say, some statement such as 'Volcanoes exist.'

In this context it is well worth remembering that for C. G. Jung and those who accept his psychological teachings psychic truths are of such a nature that they affect each and every aspect of our daily lives, meaning, for example, that historical personalities still live in the minds of each human being. From this point of view not just the teachings of such men as Paracelsus, Goethe and Rudolf Steiner, *but those men themselves*, are still alive in the minds of men and women, and any individual human being can contact them, if he or she so wishes, by travelling into the depths of inner space and bringing forth the Unconscious into full consciousness. For me at least it is difficult to believe that the person who does this, whether the techniques used are either those developed by analytical psychologists or by those associated with traditional symbol systems such as ritual magic, is not using processes similar in essence to the Imagination, Inspiration and Intuition of anthroposophical theory. It may be, of course, that the methods of developing these higher modes of perception which were advocated by Rudolf Steiner are psychologically safer and more quickly effective than those used by, for example, Jungian psychologists and practitioners of Taoist meditation; but it seems impossible, logically, to argue that the end results of the employment of any of these techniques are qualitatively different from the others.

Rudolf Steiner was, of course, only acquainted with Jung's earlier writings and it is therefore not altogether surprising that he failed to discern that there was no real incompatibility between Jungian complex psychology and his own spiritual philosophy. Nor is it in any way remarkable that he seems to have (wrongly) assumed that the Collective Unconscious of Jung bore a resemblance to the 'instinctive unconscious biological drives' of Eduard von Hartmann. What, however, is found somewhat disconcerting by most detached observers of anthroposophical thought is that intellectual attitudes that were understandable in the year 1925 but are hardly tenable at the present day are still adhered to by at least some devotees of anthroposophical medicine.

It seems unlikely that such conservative attitudes can persist indefinitely. Certainly a number of anthroposophists seem to be quietly endeavouring to arrive at personal syntheses of Jung's depth psychology, Rudolf Steiner's cosmogony, his theoretical concepts concerning the nature of humanity and the animal, plant, and mineral kingdoms over which it has dominion, which are associated with anthroposophical medicine. Such individual syntheses usually display a certain number of common features which, on the basis of personal observation, I would characterize as follows: first, a belief that C. G. Jung was quite as concerned with the 'things of the spirit' as was Rudolf Steiner. Secondly, a belief that the Collective Unconscious of Jungian depth psychology cannot be identified with the 'biological unconscious' of the pessimistic philosophy of Eduard von Hartmann but is no more than a new name for a very old occult concept, *Anima mundi*, the Soul of the World, the stored up 'spiritual treasure chest' of mankind's religious and artistic achievements and yearnings. And, finally, that Steiner's cosmogony and history, with its Crystal Heaven, its Old Saturn, its Lemuria and Atlantis, is a psychic truth in the Jungian sense, which in no way means it is not objectively true.

Whether or not personal syntheses which share the above assumptions will stand the test of the destructive criticisms of time is uncertain; what seems sure is that the formulation and critical examination of such theoretical structures indicates a surer way forward for anthroposophical devotees of holistic medicine than does a slavish adherence to the literal meaning of each and every statement made by Rudolf Steiner.

8

A Summing-up

Many physicians in general practice appear to their patients in two aspects, the healer as technologist and the healer as shaman. In the first of these medical practitioners carry out such functions as measuring blood pressure, testing urine for sugar and albumen, taking a cervical smear and so on – in other words, the physician as technologist is carrying out a series of actions which, while they may require great skill and be of great importance as aids to diagnosis and prognosis, can be learned from textbooks and are not essentially dissimilar to the diagnostic techniques employed by a motor mechanic or an electronic engineer in finding out what is wrong with a truck or a video recorder.

The shamanistic functions – I do not use the adjective in a pejorative sense – of the medical practitioner are not so easily characterized or described as those of the physician as technologist. At their lowest level they are concerned with what is still sometimes called 'the bedside manner', the capacity to create confidence and a will to recovery in the patient; at their highest they are manifested in a seemingly almost magical power of diagnosis, largely independent of technological aids, and sometimes as a capacity to heal the patient which seems totally divorced from the nature of the therapy which is prescribed. This latter capacity is indeed rare, but there is a good deal of anecdotal evidence, reminiscent of that associated with the spontaneous 'miracle cures' which are believed to take place at some Christian shrines, that some gifted physicians possess it. Jung, a qualified physician, was well aware of the fact that some medical practitioners are more successful – both financially and therapeutically – than others because they are shamans as well as technologists. He wrote: 'We must rate those doctors wise – worldly wise in every sense – who know how to surround themselves with the aura of the medicine man. They not only have the biggest practices, but also get the best results.' It is clear that Jung was not using the phrase 'medicine man' (shaman) in a denigratory sense – he was surely conscious that for his pupils and many of his patients he himself was the supreme shaman, a healer who, while employing some of the allegedly 'scientific' methods of the Freudians to bring to the surface the content of the Unconscious, interpreted that content in terms of the ideas associated with traditional mysticism and the occult.

Any man or woman who endeavours to practise holistic medicine, to treat the patient on all levels of being, physical, emotional, intellectual and spiritual, must be to some extent a shaman, a medicine man, a priest. For while it is possible for such a practitioner to use all the technological aids to diagnosis with which modern physics and chemistry have provided medicine, these will only indicate the purely physiological aspects of a patient's condition. To arrive at an understanding of the psychic and spiritual factors which may be involved, the practitioner has to act, consciously or unconsciously, as a shaman – to use some faculty (it can be dubbed 'hunch', 'sixth sense', 'clairvoyance' or 'intuition') which seemingly enables him or her, firstly, to discern the emotional and spiritual dimensions of a particular patient's illness and, secondly, to prescribe the therapy or the combination of therapies which is suitable for that patient.

There is no doubt that this shamanistic faculty is one with which some holistic physicians are more richly endowed than others. Two homoeopathic practitioners can have qualified in both orthodox medicine and homoeopathy at much the same time and, since then, have practised in a very similar way – but one will be much more successful than the other, with a reputation, spread by word of mouth, that he has a genius for curing or relieving chronic complaints which have in the past responded to neither orthodox nor alternative therapies. In the words of Jung, such a physician 'surrounds himself with the aura of the medicine man'. That is to say, those who seek his or her aid may discern a numinous quality – a 'healing virtue' – in that physician and are predisposed to benefit from his or her ministrations, because they have been imbued with a 'will to recovery'. If one wishes to use the terminology of depth psychology one can label this process of induction of the will to recovery through a belief in the healer's shamanistic powers as 'transference', but to do so in no way invalidates the process itself nor reduces the very real benefits which are experienced by the patient.

A frequent characteristic of such charismatic healers – 'charismatic' in the original sense of that word – is that the therapies they successfully prescribe are unorthodox in even the terms of their own medical unorthodoxy, homoeopathic or otherwise. Thus, for example, a homoeopathic practitioner may prescribe a potentized medicine the use of which cannot be satisfactorily accounted for on either the 'like cures like' principle or even on a vague description of the patient as being the 'such-and-such a medicine type'. And yet, in spite of the seeming irrationality of the prescription within even the half-magical context of homoeopathic principle, the remedy seems to work, the patient's disease either being alleviated or cured.

It is easy enough to say that this satisfactory outcome of treatment is 'psychological', the product of the placebo effect (see p. 63), the placebo in this case being not only the prescribed remedy but the patient's confidence in the physician. Frequently, however, particularly in such chronic diseases as dermatoses, allergies, backache, etc., the patient has been previously treated with orthodox drugs by hospital consultants, in both of which he or she had every confidence, with no benefit whatsoever – in other words, no placebo effect was discernible. Why, then, should the success of the homoeopathic 'medicine man' be attributed to the placebo effect?

If the placebo effect cannot be used to explain the success of the 'shamanistic' homoeopath or the practitioner of other varieties of holistic medicine, what can? It may be that some intrinsic healing power, of the same nature as the subtle energies or influences associated with spiritual healing, flows from or through the healer to the patient. It is likely, however, that a second and more important factor is involved: when the shaman practitioner, qualified or unqualified, successfully prescribes a homoeopathic remedy which is seemingly inappropriate to the patient's condition, or employs a particular manipulation which is unorthodox by the standards of osteopathy or chiropractice, or recommends a diet which 'doesn't make sense', he or she is actually prescribing on the basis of psychic insights, derived from some sort of hereditary or developed clairvoyance, which have indicated more surely than any cook-book rules the appropriate course of therapeutic action. In this connection it is perhaps worth remembering the intermittent but frequent success of the American seer Edgar Cayce in prescribing, while in a state of trance or semi-trance, for those who consulted him. In spite of the surprising nature of some of the 'medicines' prescribed by Cayce – they included herbs not normally considered to have any therapeutic virtues and Coca-Cola – a remarkably high proportion of his patients seem to have benefited from his eccentric ministrations. Cayce usually began his trance prescription with some such phrase as 'this body requires' or 'this being requires'. In other words, he was prescribing for a *unique* individual. Very few of Cayce's psychic prescriptions, thousands of which were recorded, are exactly the same.

It is probable that Rudolf Steiner and students of his teachings are right in believing that the trance clairvoyance of the sort exhibited by Edgar Cayce is of a primitive nature, a hangover from an earlier stage of evolution, and that as the centuries have passed this type of psychicism has become more and more prone to error, less and less appropriate to the present stage of the spiritual evolution of mankind. It seems equally likely that the same is true of the shamanistic insights of the successful healer, qualified or unqualified. This does not alter the fact that the patient benefits from such insights and that the holistic practitioner endowed with the ability to obtain them would be foolish to disregard them or abandon their use unless something better is available to replace them.

If the anthroposophists are right in what they believe, then that 'something better' has been available to the physician for over half a century – the body of theory and technique which is referred to as anthroposophical medicine. This, as has been explained in previous chapters, has been developed on the basis of authoritative indications given by Rudolf Steiner, indications which Steiner is believed to have been able to give as a result of his acquisition of knowledge derived from the employment of the supernormal modes of perception termed Imagination, Inspiration and Intuition. It is possible, so it is claimed, to develop the power to use these ways of apprehending and comprehending the realities which lie beneath physical appearances by the use of the psychic and spiritual exercises which Rudolf Steiner taught his pupils and details of at least some of which are available to anyone who cares to acquire a copy of such a book as Steiner's *Knowledge of Higher Worlds*.

It is clear that the anthroposophical physician who has acquired, however imperfectly, the ability consciously to use these higher faculties has at his or her disposal an aid to diagnosis and prescription which is immeasurably superior to that instinctive and primitive clairvoyance which is employed by at least some shamanistic healers. In addition to this, to such a physician are available both a wealth of medical teaching given by Steiner himself and a great deal of information, derived from clinical records and anthroposophical medical research, which has accumulated over the past sixty years or so. This body of stored-up anthroposophical medical wisdom makes it possible for the physician who has not yet developed the ability to use higher modes of perception, or has only developed it to a very slight extent, to practise anthroposophical medicine, to apply the insights of Rudolf Steiner and the riches of anthroposophical research and clinical experience in order to extend his or her own capacities as a healer.

Nevertheless, it is not altogether easy for the qualified physician to employ fully the medical applications of anthroposophy in the everyday activities of a practice. For, quite apart from the fact that the use of anthroposophical techniques may gain the individual practitioner a reputation for eccentricity amongst his colleagues, the anthroposophical physician has to give far more time to each individual patient than does the ordinary medical practitioner.

In *Work Arising from the Life of Rudolf Steiner* the anthroposophical physician Michael Evans has given some indications of the amount of work in which the practitioner who wishes to extend the art of healing in accordance with the principles of Rudolf Steiner is necessarily involved. He takes as an example the case of a patient suffering from Graves's disease, an overdeveloped and excessively active thyroid gland resulting in symptoms of thyrotoxicosis such as restlessness, outbursts of ill temper, an increased heart rate and so on. While, Dr Evans has explained, the proximate cause of these symptoms is undoubtedly an excessive production of thyrotoxine, the anthroposophical physician endeavours to understand what has led to the thyroid gland's overactivity. The goggle eyes which are symptomatic of Graves's disease may remind the physician of the appearance of some animal, such as a rabbit or a cat, made rigid with fright. Perhaps, such a physician might ask, the characteristic irritability of a victim of Graves's disease is also somewhat animal, an unthinking reflex response to stimuli, and perhaps the real cause of thyroid overactivity is a sort of failure to be properly human. The practitioner may then turn to some of the medical writings of Rudolf Steiner to see if he gave any indications, derived from the use of advanced modes of perception, of the subtle, that is, non-physical, factors involved in the patient's condition. Steiner did, in fact, assert that Graves's disease is associated with an astral rigidity which dominates the organism as a whole, resulting in the Ego not being in control of the emotional (astral) life of the individual. This, of course, means that the patient has reverted, in a sense, to the condition of an animal which, as it does not possess an Ego, has an emotional life which is dominated by the reflex activities of its astral body. The anthroposophical physician who has at his or her disposal all this information, derived from both direct observation of the clinical phenomena and Steiner's indications, is in a much better position, so it is asserted, to form a meaningful understanding of Graves's disease and to prescribe the appropriate remedies *for the particular patient affected by it* than is an orthodox colleague, concerned with only the physical aspects of the disease.

The therapies referred to above might include some or all of those which are standard in orthodox medicine, such as the use of drugs which reduce thyroid function or even surgical intervention, the removal of part of the gland. But it is likely that such fairly drastic measures would not be taken until the anthroposophical physician had first tried to deal with what is believed to be the cause of the disease, the rigidity and independence from the control of the Ego of the astral body, by means of holistic therapy. This may include warm baths – heat is the great stimulator of the Ego which has a relationship with elemental Fire; the subcutaneous injection of certain homoeopathic remedies[1] which, in very high potentization, are believed to influence the linkings between a human Ego and its astral vehicle; eurhythmy; and remedial massage. Some anthroposophical physicians may even employ vegetotherapy, a form of deep and almost violent massage devised by the late Wilhelm Reich which is believed to break down the variety of physical rigidity referred to as 'muscular armouring',[2] perhaps in tandem with some form of syncretistic depth analysis largely, but not entirely, derived from C. G. Jung. Even if orthodox therapies involving the administration of thyroid-immobilizing drugs and/or surgery are thought appropriate to a particular patient by an anthroposophical physician, they will almost certainly be accompanied by at least some of the holistic therapies outlined above.

A somewhat similar, although not identical, combination of holistic therapies may be considered appropriate for a very large number of 'physical' disorders, all of which are thought by the anthroposophist to involve to at least some extent the Ego and the astral and etheric bodies. Thus, for example, in certain European clinics under anthroposophical medical direction a holistic cancer therapy is practised which involves the use of eurhythmy, remedial baths and massage, painting and so on, in combination with the administration of Iscador (see p. 70) and orthodox treatments involving surgery and radiotherapy.

Provided that anthroposophical physicians avoid the 'intellectual sclerosis' which a 'Steiner and Steiner only' attitude would perhaps indicate, and provided that they are prepared to use the methods of Steiner to evaluate holistic techniques which have evolved outside an anthroposophical environment, such as vegetotherapy and depth psychology, then anthroposophical medicine may in the future develop into an holistic system which unifies orthodox and complementary medicine into a new synthesis in which the whole is greater than the sum of the parts.

APPENDIX I

Rudolf Steiner, Two English Doctors and the Origins of Anthroposophical Medicine

Various schools of holistic medicine have clearly exerted an influence upon, and contributed to, the development of anthroposophical medicine. Notable amongst these are the spagyric Paracelsian healing system, which survived the ultra-rationalist epoch of nineteenth-century medical reductionism and has enjoyed a shadowy existence until the present day, and the homoeopathy and, more particularly, the pharmacology of potentization (dynamization) developed by Samuel Hahnemann almost two centuries ago.

Nevertheless, it is generally assumed that anthroposophical medicine as such, that is, an extension of the art of healing on the basis of indications given by Rudolf Steiner, only dates from 1920, the year in which Steiner delivered his first lecture course to a specifically medical audience. It seems to me, however, that it is likely that Rudolf Steiner was not only giving medical advice well before this date, but that therapies devised by him were being administered to patients in various parts of Germany and Austria before 1912.

The diary of Franz Kafka, who certainly flirted with anthroposophy to the extent of having a personal interview with Steiner, has some significance in this connection:

The lady's doctor, when the first signs of influenza appeared in her, asked Dr Steiner for a remedy, . . . prescribed this for the lady, and restored her to health with it immediately. . . . A Munich doctor cures people with colours decided upon by Dr Steiner. He also sends invalids to the art gallery with instructions to concentrate for half an hour or longer on a particular painting.

This diary entry dates from 1911; unsupported it might mean no more than that Franz Kafka was indulging in heavy irony at Steiner's expense, as much or as little worthy of credence as Kafka's statement that Rudolf Steiner ate two litres of emulsified nuts every day. However, the diary entry must be considered in relation to a very curious statement which was in 1916 printed in the second edition of a slim English booklet entitled *Data towards the History of the Rosicrucians*:

The revived Rosicrucian Lodges on the Continent of Europe are carried on with great privacy, and their members do not openly confess to their admission and membership. Several centres are in active work under conditions derived from previous centuries of usefulness. While studying and teaching theories of life and duties and admitting members by ceremonial and ritual, many groups of the Continental Rosicrucians are, as formerly, of both sexes, and so are not necessarily Freemasons. As in the earliest times the Rosicrucians not only studied, but went about doing good and healing the sick and diseased, so now the Fratres of to-day are concerned in the study and administration of medicines, and in their manufacture upon old lines; *they also teach and practise* the curative effects of coloured light [my emphasis], and cultivate mental processes which are believed to induce spiritual enlightenment and extended powers of the human senses.

While the edition of *Data* from which the above passage has been quoted came out in 1916 its references to 'Continental Rosicrucians' must have related to the situation before the outbreak of war in 1914, for communications between English and European esotericists – even those who were citizens of Britain's allies – were difficult in the extreme from the summer of 1914 until at least the spring of 1919. Were the 'Continental Rosicrucians' who were described as using ceremonial and ritual the initiates of the esoteric masonic body led by Rudolf Steiner to which I have referred on p. 27 And do the words I have italicized confirm that, as Franz Kafka claimed, some sort of anthroposophical therapy involving coloured light was being practised as early as 1911? There are indications that the answer to both should be in the affirmative.

The author of *Data* was Dr W. Wynn Westcott, a distinguished pharmacologist and toxicologist who was also a dedicated occultist and Freemason – *Data* was, in fact, written for his fellow members of the Societas Rosicruciana in Anglia, the Rosicrucian Society in England, which still exists and, while it is not strictly speaking a masonic rite, has a masonic qualification for admittance.

Westcott was undoubtedly one of the earliest English admirers of Rudolf Steiner, regarding him as an undoubted initiate and opening a lecture he gave in 1913 to the London members of the Societas Rosicruciana with the words: 'The German Rosicrucian Theosophist, Rudolf Steiner, the author of several very instructive books in regard to Man's Origin, Constitution and Destiny. . . .'

Three years before the second edition of *Data* Westcott had produced a privately printed essay entitled *The Rosicrucians, Past and Present*, a passage in which makes it seem extremely likely that the 'Continental Rosicrucians', to whom he later referred as manufacturing medicines 'on old lines' and practising colour therapy, were indeed followers of Rudolf Steiner. Westcott wrote:

The German Rosicrucians keep their Colleges and membership entirely secret, they print no transactions nor even any notices, and it is almost impossible to identify any member.

The German groups of Rosicrucians now existing are much more immersed in mystic and occult lore than ourselves; they endeavour to extend the human faculties beyond the material towards the ethereal, astral and spiritual worlds; at the present time I understand they use no formulated Ritual, but give *vive voce* teaching, instead of written knowledge. The German Colleges have experienced a notable revival since 1900, *and the teachings of Rudolf Steiner are considered as giving an introduction to their system of occult Theosophy* [my emphasis].

This seems fairly conclusive, and assurance is strengthened by a passage in a lecture given by Westcott in 1917:

The poet Goethe, author of the drama of *Faust*, and the philosopher Leibnitz were under Rosicrucian influence. . . . They [the Rosicrucians] are in part now represented by a notable philosopher, author of many treatises on Theosophy and Anthroposophy and the Occult Sciences, Rudolf Steiner, who has several thousand pupils on the continent of Europe. From these students, modern Continental teachers who claim to be representatives of the older Rosicrucians, seek for initiates for their special culture, which leads, as they allege, to the evolution of the finer human faculties.

At the time the information given in the above quotations must have been acquired by Westcott – that is, before August 1914 – the only Rosicrucian organization in continental Europe which seems likely to have considered the teachings of Rudolf Steiner as 'an introduction to their system of occult Theosophy' was the esoteric masonry of Mysteria Maxima Aeterna (see p. 27) led by Steiner himself. It follows that the 'Continental Rosicrucians' of the passage I quote from *Data* – the adepts who are described as being 'concerned in the study and administration of medicines, and their manufacture upon old lines' – belonged to the same body and that some variety of anthroposophical medicine was being practised well before 1914.

Only one thing is against the identification of the medical Rosicrucians of the quotation from *Data* and the unquestionably anthroposophical Rosicrucians referred to in my subsequent quotations. This is the fact that the first are said to admit members by 'ceremonial and ritual', while the second are specifically described as using 'no formulated Ritual'. However, the 'no formulated Ritual' quotation dates from 1913; it seems almost certain that between then and the publication of *Data* in 1916 Westcott had acquired further information. What or who was the source of Westcott's new knowledge is not beyond the reach of all conjecture, and it seems likely to me that it was Dr R. W. Felkin, a pioneer of tropical medicine, a friend and masonic associate of Westcott, who provided the information.

Dr Felkin was the chief of a small quasi-Rosicrucian society known as the Stella Matutina, the Star of the Dawn, which was a schismatic derivative of the Hermetic Order of the Golden Dawn, which had been founded in 1888 by Westcott and others on the basis of a charter allegedly derived from continental Rosicrucians. For reasons which lie outside the scope of this book, Dr Felkin was extremely anxious to make contact with the Rosicrucians from whom, so he believed, he ultimately derived his authority as chief of the Stella Matutina. To this end he made numerous visits to Germany, seeking, as it were, a Master or Masters, and in July or August 1910 had a meeting with Rudolf Steiner. Deciding that it was at least possible that Rudolf Steiner was either a genuine Rosicrucian or, at any rate, a man who was in touch with genuine Rosicrucians, Felkin dispatched a high-grade initiate of his own order, a certain Neville Meakin, to Berlin in order to study Steiner's teachings and, perhaps, to establish some sort of link between the Stella Matutina and what Westcott was later to refer to as Rosicrucian Theosophy.

Rudolf Steiner seems to have accepted Meakin as a personal pupil, possibly on the basis of the recommendation of Baron Walleen, a Danish nobleman who was close to Steiner at the time and, interestingly enough, had at one time been an initiate of the order from which Dr Felkin's Stella Matutina was derived. At about the same time two of the earliest Englishmen to accept Steiner's teachings, Mr Harry Collison and Mr Sandrieux, were admitted into the Stella Matutina. It seems that at about this time there were tentative plans to establish a working lodge of Rudolf Steiner's 'esoteric masonry', that is Mysteria Mystica Aeterna, in England, for it is difficult to understand the contents of a letter sent by Neville Meakin of the Stella Matutina to Baron Walleen, undoubtedly an 'esoteric mason', on any other interpretation. The relevant parts of this letter read:

. . . Now I come to the Freemasonic point.

Here I tread on very delicate ground. But I feel that I must state the case, as I said, without fear or favour. The Doctor [Rudolf Steiner] is too great a man to be vexed with me. After all, all I wish to do is to secure that the best teaching reaches those most fit for it in the easiest way.

At present to establish a definite branch of the Continental Order giving grades, etc. in England will be a very difficult matter. You are not yourself a Freemason. We sometimes call our Order, the Continental Order, *Esoteric Masonry*. The grades are closely akin to Freemasonry. Dr S[teiner] indeed has some link with certain

English or Scotch Masons – he gave me the name, from whom he derives a certain authority, a link in the physical [as distinct from an 'astral link'].

. . . English Masonry boasts the Grand Lodge of 1717. . . . They are a proud, jealous, autocratic body. . . . Now the Masons who gave Dr S[teiner] his link are regarded – you had better get Dr F[elkin] to verify me here – as eccentrics who invent spurious grades. If the English Grand Lodge hears of anything called 'Esoteric Masonry', derived from such sources . . . under a head in Berlin, it will not enquire who Dr S[teiner] is or what is the nature of his work; it will simply say 'no English Masons . . . may join any society working pseudo-Masonic Rites'. . . .

Then we who are members of Dr S[teiner]'s Lodge and who are Freemasons will be in a sad plight. At present this would affect only myself, well, and Dr F[elkin] too. But if esoteric masonry is breathed of in England, and the fiat goes against it, no English Mason will wish to join the BUND [by the BUND Meakin seems to indicate the public Anthroposophical Society as distinct from semi-secret esoteric masonry].

. . . Let Messrs S[andrieux] and C[ollison] get all the MSS they can and let them establish relations with members of Hermetic Orders and Freemasons. Either let them supply such written teachings as can be given to the heads of the Lodges that will come in, and seek no interference with the Lodges, or let them form a definite committee under Dr S[teiner] with representative people in it. All this must be done slowly.

The system of having people in the Lodges like Dr F[elkin] to teach 'processes' . . . is the most practical . . . and to have . . . Messrs S[andrieux] and C[ollison] . . . to go between England and the Continent, and to get the written teaching will probably work well enough.

But if a Lodge of the Continental Order is to be established in England, Dr S[teiner] will be faced with the Masonic difficulty. This is really serious. . . . The practical solution will be found in a compromise. If he [Rudolf Steiner] avoids the name 'Esoteric Masonry' and allows perhaps a ritual like those used in the Societas Rosicruciana and the S[tella]M[atutina], and has for officers in England a mixed group, including the Heads of the chief Hermetic Lodges . . . it will succeed. Otherwise, I fear much that only a few T[heosophical] S[ociety] and a few whom Dr F[elkin] and myself . . . can influence directly, will be all that will join. . . . a foreign intrusive Masonic schism . . . will arouse every possible English prejudice against it.

Neville Meakin, the writer of the above letter, died shortly after sending it. His advice, however, was at least partly followed by Rudolf Steiner and his associates, for there is no evidence at all that a lodge of what Meakin called 'Esoteric Masonry', the Mysteria Mystica Aeterna, was ever established in Britain.

At around the time that Meakin's letter was written Dr Felkin and his wife made an extended visit to Germany in the course of which they were certainly admitted to ceremonial workings of a lodge, or lodges, of Mysteria Mystica Aeterna. There is, however, a conflict of evidence as to whether or not they were formally initiated into this order or whether they were simply allowed to see others initiated into it. There is no doubt that Dr Felkin specifically claimed that such initiations had been conferred on himself and Mrs Felkin, for in the MS 'History Lecture' of the Stella Matutina he wrote:

In June and July 1912 Frater F.R. [these initials are those of the Latin phrase *Finem respice*, 'Look to the end', which was the motto of Dr Felkin in his capacity as leader of the Stella Matutina] and Soror Q.L. [Mrs Felkin, *Quaestor lucis*] were able to go to Germany and altogether visited five Rosicrucian Temples in different parts of the Continent, and *were initiated themselves* [my emphasis], Soror Q.L. obtaining grades equivalent to our 7 = 4 [the 'Exempt Adept' grade of the Stella Matutina] and Frater F.R. 8 = 3 (the 'Master of the Temple' grade of the Stella Matutina].

The 'five Rosicrucian Temples' which Dr Felkin said he had visited were almost certainly lodges of Mysteria Mystica Aeterna and not all of them were necessarily in Germany. By this time there seem to have been established lodges of 'esoteric masonry' in Holland, Switzerland and, possibly, Italy. In this connection it is interesting to note that in the same 'History Lecture' quoted above, which Dr Felkin compiled shortly after his visit to Germany in the summer of 1912, it was stated that:

an arrangement has been come to whereby anyone conversant with German, French, Italian or Dutch, who is full 5 = 6 [the Stella Matutina's 'Minor Adept' grade], may be sent abroad with an introduction signed by F.R., and should it be considered that a candidate is sufficiently developed, one or more grades may be given him.

Dr Felkin's claim to have been ritually initiated into 'esoteric masonry' was, however, contradicted by A. E. Waite, who in his autobiography, *Shadows of Life and Thought* (Selwyn & Blount, 1938), recorded that in the course of a meeting with Rudolf Steiner he had been told that Dr Felkin had merely 'witnessed certain things – no matter what they were – of a ceremonial kind'.

Waite's statement would seem to be confirmed by a report of an interview with Rudolf Steiner which took place in March 1921. According to this,

Dr Felkin was anxious to get a charter from Dr Steiner and made many attempts to gain this and be appointed his sole representative in England. Dr Steiner, in a letter to Dr Felkin, of which I [the writer of the report] was the bearer and which I read, said he was unable to grant this request, for although ready to admit that Dr Felkin's Order was beneficial and useful, his way of working was quite different. . . . Dr Felkin was a spectator at one of Dr Steiner's ceremonies in Munich. *No grades were given him by Dr Steiner, no grades given him in Munich* [my emphasis], but Dr Steiner gave Dr Felkin a great deal of instruction.

It is possible to reconcile the conflict of evidence between Dr Felkin, writing in 1912, and Rudolf Steiner, being interviewed in 1921, on only two suppositions. First, that Dr Felkin and his wife were admitted to the rites of esoteric masonry as mere spectators and, by some extraordinary misunderstanding, believed that they had received ritual initiations of one sort or another. This seems unlikely. Felkin had been a member of various societies employing ritual for many years and he would have had to have been in a very curious state of mind to have been unable to distinguish between a ceremony in which he was a candidate for admission and one which he was merely watching. It is also intrinsically improbable that an outsider would have been admitted to the rites of a masonic or quasi-masonic body as a spectator.

The second possibility is that while, as Rudolf Steiner is reported to have said in March 1921, no grades were given by him to Felkin and no grades were conferred on Felkin in Munich, Dr and Mrs Felkin had been initiated into Mysteria Mystica Aeterna in some lodge other than Munich by some person other than Rudolf Steiner. In this connection it is perhaps significant that Felkin claimed to have visited *five* European Rosicrucian Temples, which means four temples other than Munich.

The only other possibilities are that either Dr Felkin or Rudolf Steiner was lying. Both seem unlikely.

Whatever the truth of this particular matter, whether or not Felkin was initiated into the ritual-symbolic workings of the quasi-masonic body which Rudolf Steiner closed down in 1914, there is no doubt at all that Dr Felkin was a devoted admirer of Steiner's teachings and, in due course, an active anthroposophist. It was he and his closest associates who were largely responsible for introducing anthroposophical teachings to New Zealand, to which country he permanently emigrated in 1916, setting up home at Havelock North. Here, too, he established a 'temple' of Stella Matutina, which I understand still survives, although I have no reason to believe that any of its members at the present time are also members of the Anthroposophical Society. It is interesting to note, however, that Havelock North continues to have some associations with anthroposophy and that Weleda New Zealand Ltd, an anthroposophical pharmaceutical company, has its postal address there.

It seems to me very probable that it was from Dr Felkin that Dr W. Wynn Westcott acquired his knowledge of pre-1914 'Continental Rosicrucians' who practised the healing arts and prepared medicines 'on old lines' and that these Rosicrucians were medical and other pupils of Rudolf Steiner. I conclude that some form of anthroposophical medicine of some sort was being practised, although not publicized, well before 1920, the year in which this system of holistic therapy is generally assumed to have had its beginnings.

APPENDIX II

Biodynamic Agriculture and Anthroposophical Pharmacy

Cultivated plants used in the manufacture of anthroposophic medicines are, as was explained on p. 70, almost always sown, grown and harvested in accordance with the principles of the biodynamic system of gardening and agriculture. This system, still in process of development, had its origins in the years 1922–23 when several individuals and groups approached Rudolf Steiner in order to ask his advice on problems concerned with plant and animal husbandry. He was asked, for example, about a supposed decline in the nutritional value of food, about animal sterility, and about the etheric formative forces and their connection, if any, with plant disease.

Steiner replied that plants, and the animals which were fed upon these plants, were unable to resist disease because something was wrong with their physical environment, notably the earth in which the plants were grown. It was really the soil that was sick, and that sickness had resulted from treating it as an inert mass of chemicals, suitable for dosing with nitrates, phosphates and potassium compounds, instead of as a living ecosystem with which the farmer or gardener must cooperate.

In spite of the claims he made that he had direct access to spiritual realities, that he had available other modes of perception than those of the senses, Steiner was an immensely practical man. He explained that the use of certain natural preparations, employed in conjunction with compost and farmyard manure, would be of great help in restoring vigorous life to depleted soils. These, he said, would have to be prepared by exposure 'to the rhythms of the cosmic and terrestrial forces in summer and winter', thus concentrating and enriching beneficial forces. He also gave indications for the preparation of mixtures designed to be spread directly on the soil.

In the autumn of 1922 various substances were mixed together in accordance with Steiner's suggestions and placed in somewhat unlikely containers, the horns of defunct cattle, and buried in the garden at Arlesheim, there to remain while solar, lunar and terrestrial forces supposedly exerted their influence upon them. They were dug up in the Spring with some difficulty – it had been forgotten exactly where they were buried – Steiner extracted the contents, added them to a bucket of water, stirring it with a walking stick belonging to his pupil Ehrenfried Pfeiffer, indicated how the diluted preparation should be used, and hurried away to an appointment.[1] From such casual and unpromising beginnings arose the biodynamic movement which has exerted an influence extending far beyond the limited confines of the membership of the Anthroposophical Society.

The word 'biodynamic' was not, in fact, coined by Rudolf Steiner nor does it seem to have been used by him. None the less, it accurately expresses the nature of the principles which he taught were properly applicable to all agricultural enterprise, large or small. Farming and gardening, he said, must be practised both biologically and dynamically. In other words, the soil must be regarded as a living system, not as an inert aggregation of minerals containing chemical plant nutrients such as nitrogen, phosphates and potassium; and to that soil must be applied dynamic methods, similar to those involved in the production of anthroposophic remedies, which would 'direct the flow' of seasonal, lunar and other cosmic influences.

The purely biological aspects of the biodynamic approach to agriculture, revolutionary when Steiner first formulated them, have now won considerable acceptance and are enthusiastically advocated by partisans of the worldwide ecological movement, although it seems likely that few of them appreciate to what an extent the movement was anticipated, over sixty years ago, by Rudolf Steiner. The dynamic aspect of anthroposophical agricultural theories is much less widely accepted, and few save convinced anthroposophists practise the biodynamic system in its entirety. Those who follow the whole system, whether or not they accept some of the supposed 'mystical theory' associated with it, aver that it *works*, that, judged by purely empirical standards, it gives better results than less complex organic methods of farming and gardening.

In the gardens of those companies which manufacture anthroposophic remedies, of which the Weleda group is the largest, between two and three hundred varieties of plants are cultivated in accordance with biodynamic principles. The soil is fertilized with an organic compost, compounded from animal dung and plant residues, which has been dynamized with herbal preparations derived from such sources as yarrow, nettle, dandelion and oak bark. Similarly dynamizing substances, known as preparations 500 and 501, are sprayed directly on the soil which, should its structure and composition make it desirable, is 'sweetened' with triturated coral and 'warmed' with volcanic dust.

The use of chemically synthesized pesticides and similar products is carefully avoided and biological pest controls, such as the ladybirds which prey upon aphids, are encouraged. Should these prove inadequate they are supplemented by the use of natural products which are subject to biological degradation and do not leave harmful residues in the soil; such products include derris, pyrethrum and rhyania, and, provided that the last spraying with these is done some four to six weeks before harvesting, there is little, if any, possibility that the crop will include any residue of these.

The growing of crops by the biodynamic techniques briefly described above is the first step in the production of many of the plant remedies which are so extensively employed in anthroposophical medicine. Cattle raised on farms run on biodyamic principles are fed, in so far as it is possible, on fodder produced in accordance with these principles. Thus, for example, pasture is regularly treated with Preparations 500 and 501. When it is absolutely essential to supplement biodynamically produced fodder with supplies obtained from elsewhere, every effort is made to ensure that they have been organically grown.

A veterinary adaptation of anthroposophical medicine is used in the treatment of sick farm animals if the services of a suitably qualified veterinary surgeon are available. Dynamized remedies, very similar to those employed in non-veterinary medicine, are frequently administered either instead of or in addition to conventional medicaments. Thus a disease of piglets commonly known in Germany as 'black tail' may be treated with dynamized silica in the tenth decimal potency.

APPENDIX III

Some Manufacturers and Distributors of Anthroposophical Prescription Medicines, Home Remedies and Toiletries

Australia

Mrs Robyn Connelly
121/1 Artarmon Road
Willoughby
New South Wales 2068

Mr Hendrik Dierich
PO Box 206
Kenmore
Queensland 4069

Mrs Ann Sutherland
31 Oxford Street
Hillcrest
South Australia 5086

Miss C. M. Macpherson
5/30 Middle Crescent
Brighton
Victoria 3186

Canada

Swiss Herbal Remedies
181 Don Park Road
Markham
Ontario L3R 1C2

Denmark
Medical products

A. S. Todin
Post Box 16
DK-6200 Aabenraa

Toiletries and bodycare preparations

Inger Korup
Nikolaj Plads 27
DK-1067 Copenhagen K

Germany

Weleda AG
Möhlerstrasse 3–5
D7070 Schwabisch Gmünd

Iceland

Mrs Hulda Jensdottir
Porfinnsgt 16
Reykjavik

Netherlands

Handelsonderneming Weleda
Van der Spiegelstraat 16
NL-2518 ET The Hague

New Zealand

Weleda New Zealand Ltd
PO Box 132
Havelock North

Norway
Medical products

NORSK Medisinaldepot
Post Box 100
N-Oslo-5

Toiletries and bodycare preparations
>Helios A/L
>Post Box 222
>N-3470 Slemmestad

Sweden
Medical products
>Stiftelsen Nordiska
>Laboratorier
>Box 48
>S-15300 Jarna

Toiletries and bodycare preparations
>Weleda AB
>Box 15108
>S-161 15 Bromma

Switzerland
>WALA-Heilmittel GMBH
>D-7327 Eckwalden/Bad Boll

>Weleda AG
>CH-4144 Arlesheim

South Africa
>Weleda SA
>PO Box 494
>ZA-2012 Bergvlei
>Transvaal

United Kingdom
>Weleda UK Ltd
>Heanor Road
>Ilkeston
>Derbyshire
>DE7 8DR

United States
>Weleda Inc.
>841 South Main Street
>Spring Valley
>NY 10977

NOTES

CHAPTER 1

1. The adjective 'anthroposophical' and the noun from which it derives seem to have evolved from the title of the Welsh writer Thomas Vaughan's *Anthroposophia Theomagica*, 1650.
2. Amongst Eckstein's associates was the youthful Sigmund Freud and there is some possibility that, through Eckstein, Theosophical ideas exerted some influence upon the development of psychoanalysis. In this connection see pp. 350–52 of the late James Webb's *The Occult Establishment*, Richard Drew, 1981.
3. The full text of the lecture, given on 25 February 1912, can most easily be found in *Psychoanalysis in the Light of Anthroposophy*, Anthroposophic Press, New York, 1946.
4. It seems possible that von Hartmann's total pessimism owed something to the fact that he endured much pain from a diseased knee. According to Steiner, this diseased knee resulted from an incident in one of von Hartmann's earlier incarnations, being the consequence of a 'karmic injustice' he had committed during the Crusades. Such remarkable statements as this have led some commentators on Steiner to have regarded him as either a hoaxer or a lunatic. Both attitudes are, I think, mistaken and I suspect that Steiner was making a statement about von Hartmann which was intended to convey a psychological truth about the inmost nature of the philosopher, not a material fact of the 1 + 1 = 2 variety.
5. See Ellic Howe, *Urania's Children*, William Kimber, 1967, p. 80.
6. The coming Christhood of Krishnamurti had been first

discovered by C. W. Leadbeater, a man who might almost be regarded as Annie Besant's evil genius and whose interest in the boy does not seem to have been exclusively Theosophical. In this connection, see Francis King, *Il Cammino del Serpente*, Edizioni Mediterranée, Rome, 1979, pp. 175–99.

7. Steiner's unusual and highly personal approach to Rosicrucianism can most easily be met with in the pages of his *Rosicrucian Esotericism*, Anthroposophic Press, New York, 1978.

8. For example, abusive pamphlets and books by Grigori Bostunitsch – a one-time admirer of Steiner who later became a member of Heinrich Himmler's SS – and Max Seiling.

9. Subsequently the OTO or, at any rate, a substantial number of its initiates came under the leadership of Aleister Crowley. The Crowleyan OTO still survies, although it is now divided into at least four competing schisms.

10. Steiner seems to have wound up his esoteric masonry in the summer of 1914.

CHAPTER 2

1. The most easily available English translation of the lecture from which this quotation has been taken is Rudolf Steiner, *The Occult Significance of Blood*, Rudolf Steiner Press, 1967.

2. A perhaps unduly literal translation of this lecture will be found in Steiner's *Psychoanalysis in the Light of Anthroposophy*, Anthroposophic Press, New York, 1946.

3. See Steiner's lecture of 2 July 1921.

4. Owing to a wobble in the earth's rotation, the position of the sun in relation to the fixed sidereal zodiac (as outlined by the constellations) at the time of the spring equinox moves backwards each year by a fraction of a degree. By convention, however, astronomers and Western astrologers *call* the moving point at which the sun is situated at the moment of the vernal equinox 'the 0 degree of Aries', although it is now many degrees from the 0 degree of the *constellation* of Aries. In a period of approximately 26,000 years the moving of 0 degree Aries makes a complete revolution of 360 degrees and once more coincides with true 0 degree Aries. This is the Great Year; it is interesting to note that the ancients, who used the pre-Julian calendar

which divided the solar year into only 360 days, talked of
a 'Great Month' of thirty 'days', equivalent to 2160 solar
years, roughly the time it takes the vernal point to travel
backwards through one sign of the zodiac. This means that
the 'Great Day', the period in which the vernal point moves
backwards by 1 degree, is of a duration of seventy-two years
– Steiner's 'ideal' human lifespan.

CHAPTER 3

1. Dynamized medicines produced by the Swiss company
   WALA contain no alcohol whatsoever.
2. In cases where the raw material is an insoluble solid the
   successive succussions with a dilutant liquid are replaced by
   repeated grindings (triturations) with a solid 'dilutant',
   usually lactose (milk sugar).
3. See: M. R. Evans and A. W. Preece, 'Viscum album – a
   possible treatment for cancer?', *Bristol Medico-Chirurgical
   Journal*, vol. 88, 1973; Michael Evans, *Extending the Art of
   Healing*, Weleda, n.d.; Victor Bott, *Anthroposophical
   Medicine*, Rudolf Steiner Press, 1978, pp. 161–80.
4. The use of such composite remedies is, of course, pure heresy
   from the point of view of classical homoeopathy, in which
   only medicines derived from single substances are employed.

CHAPTER 4

1. Anthroposophical physicians also recommend that a
   pregnant woman should endeavour to live placidly, not (in
   the words of an anonymous anthroposophist) 'bombarding
   herself with sense impressions which might adversely affect
   her unborn child'. On the face of it, this might appear a
   somewhat strange idea, but it has to be admitted that if a
   pregnant woman subjects herself to certain violent stimuli,
   for example those which lead to the production of large
   quantities of adrenaline, these might well have some influence
   on the development of the embryo.
2. In view of the substantial amount of cholesterol contained
   in eggs, and the possibility that this may result in a
   diminution in the amount of blood supplied to the brain,
   Steiner's advice may not have been as silly as Kafka clearly
   thought it to have been.
3. One is here reminded of Coleridge's son, Hartley, who

burned out young, and of the short-lived Edward VI, only son of King Henry VIII, who was reputed to have written excellent Greek verse at the age of six and was certainly dead ten years later. It is almost needless to say that not all children who are subjected to such early cramming either die young or even become intellectually burned out – Lord Macaulay provides a case in point. It does seem, however, that the products of such intensive rearing tend to be either unstable or so intellectually priggish that they are cut off from any real empathetic contact with their fellow human beings.

4. Such a combination, as Dr Victor Bott has pointed out, is to be found in some Italian spa waters. I am told that the same combination is to be found, in extreme dilution, in the springs of Hotwells, Somerset.

CHAPTER 5

1. This matter is dealt with at some length in the outline of Rudolf Steiner's cosmogony which is given in chapter 7.
2. The planet Venus and the goddess of the same name, also known as Aphrodite, have been believed to be associated with metallic copper since classical times; the very word 'copper' is derived from the name of the island of Cyprus, traditional birthplace of Aphrodite.
3. Interestingly enough, it is claimed that the process involved in the purification of some public water supplies inevitably produce a similar devitalization. For this reason some anthroposophical paediatricians have advocated that young children should be given bottled spring water, rather than tap water, to drink and should be bathed, whenever possible, in rain water.
4. For a partial listing of these, see Appendix III.

CHAPTER 6

1. Kandinsky was profoundly influenced by both Steiner's exposition of Goethe's theory of colour and the descriptions of thought forms given by H. P. Blavatsky's disciple C. W. Leadbeater.
2. A very similar process of ossification can be discerned in the history of small political parties.
3. Rudolf Steiner also taught that Karl Marx's obsessional hatred

of those who owned large amounts of private property was a karmic consequence of an event which took place in an earlier life – the seizure of his lands by a disagreeable nobleman who was later reincarnated as Friedrich Engels.

4. Some anthroposophical physicians have close connections with the Camphill Movement, as do some priests of the Christian community, the theology of which body has been much influenced by Steiner although by no means all of those who belong to it are members of the Anthroposophical Society. I understand that during Dr Konig's lifetime there was a Camphill School of Spiritual Science in which methods of attaining to supernormal modes of perception were taught, but that this has been absorbed into the similarly named school which has its headquarters at the Goetheanum.

5. The sensitivity of the dolphin's skin and the supposed polarity between skin and liver (see p. 121) is the basis for this curious suggestion.

CHAPTER 7

1. This and other quotations referring to anthroposophical cosmogony are taken from Rudolf Steiner's *Occult Science*, first published in 1910.

2. There is a specifically anthroposophical development of astrology which is termed astrosophy.

3. It is interesting to note that H. P. Blavatsky was also of this opinion, specifically stating that the aboriginal Tasmanians were of Lemurian descent.

4. Manu – an initiate who also had a certain importance in the cosmogonies expounded by occultists as various as Saint-Yves, H. P. Blavatsky and Dion Fortune.

5. Docetism is represented at the present day by Christian Science, which does indeed teach that Christ's body (like that of everybody else) was illusory.

6. 'Science', of course, in the sense in which that word was used by the translators of the Authorized Version of the Bible, i.e. as an equivalent of the Greek word *gnosis*.

7. A much lengthier schematicized account, together with some extremely useful tabulations, will be found in G. Ahern, *The Sun at Midnight* (Aquarian Press, 1981). The version of the history of mankind given by Steiner is *not* identical with that expounded by H. P. Blavatsky and her followers, but it does have certain very strong similarities. For an outline

account of Blavatskyan cosmogony/history see my *Satan and Swastika* (Granada, 1975) which also points out Blavatsky's indebtedness to earlier occult systematizers.

8. Lancelot Law Whyte has pointed out that the concept of the existence of unconscious mental processes was topical by the beginning of the nineteenth century and fashionable by 1870–80.

9. There is a curiously close, but perhaps entirely coincidental, link between Sigmund Freud and Rudolf Steiner: Joseph Breuer, Freud's friend, collaborator and, for a time, patron, seems to have been a friend of at least two families to whose children Rudolf Steiner acted as tutor.

10. It would seem that the contemporary cult of biorhythms is at least partly derived, through Fliess, from ancient numerological beliefs.

11. This was V. M. Firth, who wrote on occult matters under the pseudonym of Dion Fortune and was reputed to be an extremely powerful trance medium through whom 'the Masters' spoke. V. M. Firth, like some other early psychotherapists, such as Homer Lane, seems never to have had a training analysis. Details of her psychotherapeutic career should be contained in Alan Richardson's forthcoming biography.

CHAPTER 8

1. As the reader of this book will have appreciated, many of the remedies used by homoeopathic physicians are also employed by anthroposophical practitioners, who also use many specifically anthroposophical medicines in what is sometimes, not strictly correctly, referred to as 'homoeopathic dilution', that is in potentized form. This has led some people with a vague awareness of the existence of anthroposophical medicine to a mistaken belief that it is no more than a variant of homoeopathy. This idea is mistaken on many counts, perhaps the four most notable of them being: (a) that while the 'like cures like' principle of classical homoeopathy is regarded as being a useful indication of the possible medical value of a particular plant, animal or mineral substance, it is not regarded by the anthroposophist as being either uniquely important or always valid; (b) that by no means all anthroposophic remedies are administered in potentized form; (c) that the anthroposophical physician often administers medicines

derived from more than one source, whereas the practitioner of classical homoeopathy adheres to Hahnemann's rigid insistence that medicines should always be 'simple', derived from one substance only; and (d) that the anthroposophist applies many non-homoeopathic therapies such as eurhythmy, remedial massage and so on.

2. At least some anthroposophists think it possible that the 'orgone energy' with which Reich concerned himself was in reality astral 'substance' and that the muscular rigidity which Reich regarded as resulting from effects produced by the dammed-up forces of the libido is, in fact, a physical expression of an astral rigidity of the sort which Rudolf Steiner thought to be associated with Graves's disease.

APPENDIX II

1. See E. Pfeiffer, *Bio-Dynamic Gardening and Farming*, Mercury Press, New York, 1983.

BIBLIOGRAPHY

General introductions to anthroposophy and Rudolf Steiner's thought

The following books all provide, in their very different ways, good introductions to anthroposophy and the teachings of Rudolf Steiner. Most readers will perhaps find that Colin Wilson's book provides the most wide-ranging and readable introduction to Steiner's thought, but Dr Ahern's somewhat sociological approach to the worldwide anthroposophical movement is derived from first-hand experience and should on no account be neglected. The late Canon Shepherd's book undoubtedly appeals to those who both appreciate hagiography and have an uncritical admiration for Rudolf Steiner and all his works.

Geoffrey Ahern, *Sun at Midnight*, Aquarian Press, 1984.

A. P. Shepherd, *A Scientist of the Invisible*, Hodder & Stoughton, 1958.

Colin Wilson, *Rudolf Steiner, the Man and His Vision*, Aquarian Press, 1985.

Books of general interest in relationship to occultism and anthroposophy

Owen Barfield, *Romanticism Comes of Age*, Faber & Faber, 1944.

Owen Barfield, 'The Art of Eurhythmy', in *The Golden Blade*, Rudolf Steiner Press, 1954.

J. Darcy (ed.), *Work Arising from the Life of Rudolf Steiner*, Rudolf Steiner Press, 1975.

Ellic Howe, *The Magicians of the Golden Dawn*, Aquarian Press, 1984.

Ellic Howe, *Urania's Children,* William Kimber, 1967.

F. King, *Il Cammino del Serpente,* Edizioni Mediterranée, Rome, 1979.

F. King, *The Magical World of Aleister Crowley,* Weidenfeld & Nicolson, 1977.

K. Konig, *Rudolf Steiner's Calendar of the Soul,* Rudolf Steiner Press, n.d.

E. Pfeiffer, *Bio-Dynamic Gardening and Farming,* Mercury Press, New York, 1983.

F. Rittelmeyer, *Rudolf Steiner Enters My Life,* Christian Community Press, 1963.

Rudolf Steiner, *Christianity as Mystical Fact and the Mysteries of Antiquity,* Rudolf Steiner Press, 1972.

Rudolf Steiner, *Occult Science,* Rudolf Steiner Press, 1972.

Rudolf Steiner, *Rosicrucian Esotericism,* Anthroposophic Press, New York, 1978.

Rudolf Steiner, *Rosicrucianism and Modern Initiation,* Garden City Press, 1965.

Rudolf Steiner, *The Four Seasons and the Archangels,* Rudolf Steiner Press, 1968.

Rudolf Steiner, *Theosophy,* Kegan Paul, Trench, Trubner, 1910.

Rudolf Steiner, *The Philosophy of Freedom,* Rudolf Steiner Press, 1964.

Rudolf Steiner, *The Spiritual Hierarchies and Their Reflection in the Physical World – Zodiac, Planets, Cosmos,* Anthroposophic Press, New York, 1972.

G. Wachsmuth, *The Evolution of Mankind,* Philosophic Anthroposophic Press, Dornach, 1971.

J. Webb, *The Flight from Reason,* Macdonald, 1971.

J. Webb, *The Harmonious Circle,* Thames & Hudson, 1980.

J. Webb, *The Occult Establishment,* Richard Drew, 1981.

Books of particular relevance to anthroposophical medicine

Victor Bott, *Anthroposophical Medicine,* Rudolf Steiner Press, 1982.

Michael Evans, *Extending the Art of Healing,* Weleda UK Ltd, n.d.

N. Glas, *Conception, Birth and Early Childhood,* Anthroposophic Press, New York, 1972.

V. Grahl, *The Exceptional Child,* Rudolf Steiner Press, 1970.

M. Hauschka, *Rhythmical Massage,* Rudolf Steiner Press, 1979.

Walter Holtzapfel, *Children's Destinies*, Mercury Press, New York, 1978.

M. Kirchner-Bockholt, *Fundamentals of Curative Eurhythmy*, Rudolf Steiner Press, 1978.

R. Leroi, *An Anthroposophical Approach to Cancer*, Mercury Press, New York, 1977.

E. Pfeiffer, *Sensitive Crystallization Processes*, Anthroposophic Press, New York, 1975.

Rudolf Steiner, *Agriculture*, Bio-Dynamic Agricultural Association, 1974.

Rudolf Steiner, *Anthroposophical Approach to Medicine*, Anthroposophical Publishing Co., 1951.

Rudolf Steiner, *Curative Education*, Rudolf Steiner Press, 1972.

Rudolf Steiner, *Psychoanalysis in the Light of Anthroposophy*, Anthroposophic Press, New York, 1946.

Rudolf Steiner, *Spiritual Science and Medicine*, Rudolf Steiner Press, 1975.

Rudolf Steiner, *Spiritual Science and the Art of Healing*, Anthroposophical Publishing Co., 1950.

Rudolf Steiner, *Supersensible Man*, Anthroposophical Publishing Co., 1943.

Rudolf Steiner, *The Four Temperaments*, Anthroposophic Press, New York, 1976.

Rudolf Steiner, *The Occult Significance of Blood*, Rudolf Steiner Press, 1967.

Rudolf Steiner and Ita Wegman, *Fundamentals of Therapy*, Rudolf Steiner Press, 1967.

Otto Wolff (ed.), *The Anthroposophical Approach to Medicine*, vol. I, Anthroposophic Press, New York, 1982.

W. Zu Linden, *A Child is Born*, Rudolf Steiner Press, 1973.

Index

(Note: There are no entries in this index for references which are to be found on almost every page, such as 'Steiner, Rudolf'. In the case of phrases which recur with great frequency, such as 'rhythmic system', only major page references are given.)